PEDIATRICS, CHILD AND ADOLESCENT HEALTH

UNDERSTANDING AUTISM SPECTRUM DISORDER

CURRENT RESEARCH ASPECTS

Pediatrics, Child and Adolescent Health

Joav Merrick - Series Editor

National Institute of Child Health
and Human Development,
Ministry of Social Affairs, Jerusalem

Child and Adolescent Health Yearbook 2012
Joav Merrick (Editor)
2012. ISBN: 978-1-61942-788-4 (Hardcover)
2012. ISBN: 978-1-61942-789-1 (E-book)

Child Health and Human Development Yearbook 2011
Joav Merrick (Editor)
2012. ISBN: 978-1-61942-969-7 (Hardcover)
2012. ISBN: 978-1-61942-970-3 (E-book)

Child and Adolescent Health Yearbook 2011
Joav Merrick (Editor)
2012. ISBN: 978-1-61942-782-2 (Hardcover)
2012. ISBN: 978-1-61942-783-9 (E-book)

Tropical Pediatrics: A Public Health Concern of International Proportions
Richard R Roach, Donald E Greydanus, Dilip R Patel, Douglas N Homnick and Joav Merrick (Editors)
2012. ISBN: 978-1-61942-831-7 (Hardcover)
2012. ISBN: 978-1-61942-840-9 (E-book)

Child Health and Human Development Yearbook 2012
Joav Merrick (Editor)
2012. ISBN: 978-1-61942-978-9 (Hardcover)
2012. ISBN: 978-1-61942-979-6 (E-book)

Developmental Issues in Chinese Adolescents
Daniel TL Shek, Rachel CF Sun and Joav Merrick (Editors)
2012. ISBN: 978-1-62081-262-4 (Hardcover)
2012. ISBN: 978-1-62081-270-9 (E-book)

Positive Youth Development: Theory, Research and Application
Daniel TL Shek, Rachel CF Sun and Joav Merrick (Editors)
2012. ISBN: 978-1-62081-305-8 (Hardcover)
2012. ISBN: 978-1-62081-347-8 (E-book)

Positive Youth Development: A New School Curriculum to Tackle Adolescent Developmental Issues
Hing Keung Ma, Daniel TL Shek and Joav Merrick (Editors)
2012. ISBN: 978-1-62081-384-3 (Hardcover)
2012. ISBN: 978-1-62081-385-0 (E-book)

Transition from Pediatric to Adult Medical Care
David Wood, John G. Reiss, Maria E. Ferris, Linda R. Edwards and Joav Merrick (Editors)
2012. ISBN: 978-1-62081-409-3 (Hardcover)
2012. ISBN: 978-1-62081-412-3 (E-book)

Understanding Autism Spectrum Disorder: Current Research Aspects
Ditza A Zachor and Joav Merrick (Editors)
2012. ISBN: 978-1-62081-353-9 (Hardcover)
2012. ISBN: 978-1-62081-390-4 (E-book)

PEDIATRICS, CHILD AND ADOLESCENT HEALTH

UNDERSTANDING AUTISM SPECTRUM DISORDER

CURRENT RESEARCH ASPECTS

DITZA A ZACHOR
AND
JOAV MERRICK
EDITORS

NOVA BIOMEDICAL
New York

For permission to use material from this book please contact us:
Telephone 631-231-7269; Fax 631-231-8175
Web Site: http://www.novapublishers.com

Library of Congress Cataloging-in-Publication Data

ISBN 978-1-62081-353-9

Library of Congress Control Number: 2012934500

Published by Nova Science Publishers, Inc. † New York

Contents

Autism spectrum disorders

Ditza A Zachor, MD[1*] and Joav Merrick, MD, MMedSci, DMSc[2,3,4]

[1]The Autism Center, Child Neurology and Development Unit, Assaf Harofeh Medical Center, Zerifin, Israel, [2]National Institute of Child Health and Human Development, Office of the Medical Director, Health Services, Division for Intellectual and Developmental Disabilities,Ministry of Social Affairs and Social Services, Jerusalem, [3]Division of Pediatrics, Hadassah Hebrew University Medical Centers, Mt Scopus Campus, Jerusalem and [4]Kentucky Children's Hospital, University of Kentucky, Lexington, Kentucky, United States of America

Autism spectrum disorders (ASD) are common neurodevelopmental disorders characterized by a triad of impairments in reciprocal social interactions, verbal and non-verbal communication deficits with repetitive and stereotyped behaviors. The concept of autism spectrum accurately describes the broad continuum of variation and severity in symptomatology, ranging from mild to very severe symptoms in each of the three areas of impairments. Although the prognosis for children with ASD is variable, the disorder generally has lifelong effects on the child's ability to socialize, to care for him/her self and to participate meaningfully in the community. The disorder may adversely impact not just the affected child, but also his/her family members. Currently there is no effective means for prevention, no biomarkers for early diagnosis and no specific treatment approach or a drug that can "cure" the disorder.

Interest in ASD has exploded in the past decade following the vast increase in the prevalence of ASD to 1:100-1:150 in the most recent reports. The dramatic increase in ASD cases has been accompanied by increase in public and professional awareness and an abundance of new research and treatment strategies. What was once thought to be a rare, severe disorder is now recognized to be a common neurobehavioral disorder, which occurs along a broad continuum. Autism is probably not a single disorder, but rather reflects many different disorders with broad behavioral phenotypes causing atypical development.

* *Correspondence:* Ditza A Zachor, MD, Director, The Autism Center, Assaf HaRofeh Medical Center, Sackler School of Medicine, IL-70300 Zerifin, Israel. E-mail: dzachor@asaf.health.gov.il

The cause of autism is unknown. Evidence from twin and family studies indicates that autism is highly heritable. However, no single specific gene has been consistently identified to be playing a major role in most cases. Rather, autism is thought to involve a complex interaction between multiple and variable susceptibility genes and epigenetic effects. Although brain abnormalities in autism are complex and not consistently identified, an intriguing pattern of brain growth has been discovered that involves rapid growth of head circumference during the first 3-4 years of life that slows down later in development. Enlarged white matter, variation in myelination and impaired connectivity between brain regions were discovered and are thought to be related to functional impairments and poor information processing.

An exciting area of study involves early diagnosis of autism by characterizing early behaviors and abnormal developmental patterns that are evident well before a definite diagnosis of ASD is made. Intriguing behavioral differences in receptive and expressive language, gestures, joint attention skills, pointing, visual attention, social responsiveness and temperamental characteristics were documented as early as at 12 months between siblings later diagnosed with autism and those who do not meet criteria for diagnosis.

Early identification of ASD and early provision of treatment can improve outcomes for many affected children. Cortical plasticity during early development enables the child to acquire new skills when receiving a proper intervention leading to a better prognosis. The need for early focused intervention that will result in meaningful outcomes in cognitive, language, and adaptive skills provides a fertile ground for intervention research across many disciplines.

The majority of children with ASD will need intensive and regular therapy aimed at improving communication, socialization and behavior and to improve cognition, language and adaptive skills. Behavioral, educational and psychosocial interventions have been the cornerstone of treatment for individuals with ASD. The complexity of the disorder frequently requires complex treatment strategies, which include the integration of many treatments that are tailored to the child's needs and may need to change throughout development.

Commonly associated symptoms in autism include inattention, hyperactivity, impulsivity, aggression, self injurious behaviors, excessive compulsions, affective instability, seizures, feeding and sleep problems. In addition to behavioral intervention some of these behavioral problems respond well to drug interventions. Drug treatments when necessary, frequently enhance the person's ability to benefit from educational and psychosocial interventions and can improve the quality of life for the individual and his family.

Research has focused on early clinical detection of ASD, finding biomarkers for early and accurate diagnosis, looking for possible neurobiological etiologies, developing new treatment approaches and use of pychopharmacology.

This book on autism addresses some of these important research questions and provides comprehensive up-to-date reviews on myriad of important areas in ASD. Issues such as biological markers, dilemmas in the diagnostic process, attachment and family characteristics are discussed. This book brings descriptions of various comprehensive treatment modalities and experimental pharmacology aimed at improving core autism symptoms and complex behavior and developmental problems.

Section one: Autism spectrum disorders

In: Understanding Autism Spectrum Disorder
Editors: Ditza A Zachor and Joav Merrick

ISBN: 978-1-62081-353-9

Chapter 1

Using an ecological approach to understand perception, cognition and action coupling in individuals with autism spectrum disorder

*Amy Lynch[1] and Nancy Getchell[2]**
[1]Childrens Hospital of Philadelphia, PA
[2]Department of Kinesiology and Applied Physiology, University of Delaware, Newark, Deleware, US

Abstract

Current theoretical and empirical thought suggests that successful performance of goal-directed movements require an integration of perceptual, cognitive, and motor processes. The act of movement generates a dynamic interchange amongst the three systems: Movement yields feedback from different sensory organs, and this new information must be integrated and upgraded until the individual completes the movement. Both development and experience generate tighter coupling of perception, cognition, and action, leading to less variability in performance and increased efficiency of movements, which adequately support actions that are more skilled. For children Autism Spectrum Disorder (ASD), one or several processes may be deficient along the sequence from perception to action. This may generate persistent variability and challenge ideal motor performance for success in daily activities. Although the body of research is relatively small, researchers whose studies examine motor functioning in children with ASD generally conclude that motor deficiencies exist across a range of skills, including fine and gross motor domains such as posture, balance, and locomotion. However, there remains a question related to the nature of these impairments: Where within the process of perception-cognition-action coupling do children with ASD differ from typically developing children? In this chapter, we review both theory and research related to the

* Correspondence: Nancy Getchell, Department of Kinesiology and Applied Physiology, 157 Rust Ice Arena, University of Delaware, Newark, DE 19716 United States. Tel: (302) 831-6682; Fax: (302) 831-3693; E-mail: getchell@udel.edu.

process of perception-cognition-action coupling in children with ASD in a heuristic attempt to stimulate new types of empirical studies. The discussion is framed within an ecological perspective.

Introduction

Clinicians and clinical based authors propose that motor, sensory, and behavioral impairments exist within children with autism. While numerous theories and interventions propose to address the behavioral challenges, researchers aiming to quantify motor impairments in support of evidence based practice face methodological issues due in large part to the sensory and behavioral characteristics. Interestingly, the motor impairments of children with autism which are not included as diagnostic criteria in either the Diagnostic Statistics Manual of Disorders (1) nor in the International Classifications of Diseases (2). The clearest behavioral impairments, such as issues with communication, social relationships, and imaginative thought (1), in conjunction with sensory processing impairments may negatively impact research participation as a result of decreased comprehension of tasks, motivation, and/or attention to task completion. This challenges researchers who aim to systematically describe the motor deficits impacting daily function for children with autism.

Despite the lack of inclusion of motor impairment as diagnostic criterion for ASD, a growing body of research has evolved surrounding the issue. Researchers have found that individuals with ASD move differently than typically developing children (3-5). To date, however, researchers have not adopted a theoretical paradigm that directs both thought and study of ASD in respect to motor performance. In this regard, we suggest that adoption of an ecological perspective may aid in both understanding the relationship amongst perception, cognition, and action as they contributes motor control and coordination issues in people with ASD.

Emerging research suggests that individuals with ASD have impairments across various systems, including sensory perception, cognition, and motor. Individuals with ASD often show sensory perceptual processing dysfunction, which in turn, may impede successful and meaningful sensory motor activity as well as cognitive learning (6,7). Cognitive and perceptual impairments may exist at processing levels (8), such as the integration and use of contextual sensory information (9), categorization skills of object qualities and object use/knowledge (10,11), and attention (13). Self-generated motor action by these children, represented by motor execution and activity performance, exhibit difficulty with timing, sequencing, initiation, and force control (13-15). In addition, children also demonstrate impairments in imitation motor actions (16-17). Thus, in isolation, the categories of perception, cognition, and action impairment exist in available ASD literature.

Given the challenges posed in research design for this population, it is understandable that thus far, researchers have primarily attempted to compartmentalize systems and enhance understanding of specific deficits in ASD. Few have attempted to examine the associations among them as a way to understand the 'gestalt' of ASD. Since focusing on these three systems individually (perception, cognition, action) downplays the relationships among these systems, future research to advance understanding ASD should begin with the assumption that a dynamic interdependency exists among perceptual, cognitive, and motor systems within the human body. Such an approach comes from the adoption of an Ecological perspective.

Understanding the ecological perspective

Application of ecological perspective assures consideration of the whole human system as greater than the sum of different physiological sub-systems and has been used as a premise to study individuals who are typically developing (18) as well as those with physical (19), learning (20) and developmental (21,22) disabilities. According to the theoretical framework, a child moves as a result of a dynamic interaction between perceptual, cognitive, and motor systems (23-25). Given function of children with autism is closely coupled with environmental factors, the ecological perspective that individuals cannot be understood remote from their environment (26) makes it an ideal backdrop for consideration of the motor challenges of children with ASD. In further support for the ecological perspective is the theory's shared notion of embodied cognition. As Thelen (24) suggested, "cognition depends on the kinds of experience that come from having a body with particular perceptual and motor capabilities that are inseparably linked and that together form the matrix within which reasoning, memory, emotion, language, and all other aspects of metal life are embedded (pp. 5)". This further supports an attempt to evaluate more closely the motor abilities of children with autism towards understanding the multi-system challenges posed and impacting participation in daily life.

Important features of an ecological perspective as applied to ASD

Consider the following situation. A young child is in his home, playing as he lines up trains while humming in the toy room. His parent calls him to dinner, and he leaves his toys, walks to the dining room, and sits down. If we focus on one intended action (walking), it is clear that this requires coordination among sensation, thought, and limb movement throughout the process. The child must tolerate an interruption in an already established action sequence (lining up trains), in order to register the new auditory input of the parent direction. Next, he must differentiate the parent auditory input of the words spoken to him, interpret their meaning, and plan and execute an action (halt motor activity with known play activity of trains, and initiate motor action to navigate home and walk into the kitchen). During the action, perceptual information changes which may have a profound impact on both cognition and action. More subtle perceptual, cognition, and action coupling may come into play, such as the tone of voice of the parent (angry, anxious, carefree), the physiological state of the child (sated, hungry), and the immediate environment (cluttered with toys, furniture obstacles to navigate, smells from the kitchen). For a child developing typically, the transition and underlying processing described are both seamless. For a child developing with autism, transitions are challenging, quite potentially because of impairments in the described processes. An ecological perspective suggests that, in order to understand the action seen within this scenario, one must consider the child (individual) within the immediate environment performing a specific task (27). Within this context, several key principles exist that may aid in the study of ASD.

Emergent behavior

When considering research into ASD, the principle of emergent behavior suggests that intact cognition, perception, and action systems dynamically interchange in a fashion that leads to self-organization of functional, proficient movement. In essence, behavior 'emerges' from the interaction of these systems within a context. At the same time, the dynamic interchange among these when one or more systems is impaired may lead to self-organization of maladaptive motor patterns. Furthermore, the environment in which one moves joins in the dynamic mix. In order to understand the way in which particular movement patterns naturally self-organize in individuals with ASD, one must be careful understand the important role that environment plays on behaviors Klin et al (28) discusses these phenomena:

"One of the most intriguing puzzles posed by individuals with autism is the great discrepancy between what they can do on explicit takes of social reasoning (when all of the elements of the problem are verbally given to them), and what they fail to do in more naturalistic situations (when they need to spontaneously apply their social reasoning ability it meet the moment-by-moment demands of their daily social life)". Klin et al (28) goes on to explain these phenomena through the notion of an embodied mind, imparting the salience of natural setting on resultant behaviors. The principle of self-organization is that no single system can account for all differences seen between individuals with and without ASD; rather, the interaction of these systems within a context allows adaptive behaviors to emerge.

Return to the example of the child described above, playing with a train; in this new scenario, the child has autism. His ability to perceive and integrate sensory information is impaired, so that he has difficulty selectively attending to his parent's voice over a myriad of other concurrent auditory stimuli (music, television, siblings). Further, he has difficulty coupling the sound of the voice with the meaning of the words; this may be further complicated by the parent's choice of words in which abstract ideas may not be interpreted, such as "I hope you're as hungry as a horse! " vs. a more concrete "You need to come to the table to eat dinner". Once the child interprets the parent's meaning, he must couple this to an appropriate plan of action, which may prove difficult given social communication issues. Finally, he must move, at which point, the child is once again confronted with changing sensory stimuli, which he must again interpret and modify in an effort to adapt his movements. Perceptual, cognitive, and motor systems interact throughout this entire process.

Stability, variability and change

Practitioners working with children with ASD recognize that their patients go through potentially long periods where they could not perform a skill or task, followed by periods of variegated success and failure, followed by more stable production of the action. These 'stages' of proficiency can be viewed as different 'attractor states' of the individual. In sum, there are endless combinations of degrees of freedom within the body; however, the body seems 'attracted' to a narrow range of motor behaviors. In the terms of an ecological perspective, certain 'attractor states' exist, which represent preferred, dynamically stable behaviors. If a strong attractor state exists, it is difficult to change the motor behavior. In fact, when an individual with ASD exhibits stereotypical behaviors such as hand flapping, he or she exhibits a strong, stable attractor state (generally in response to a need for sensory input to the vestibular and visual system. Another such attractor state relates to limb coordination. Limbs are most preferentially attracted to either in-phase (e.g. clapping, jumping) or anti-phase (e.g. walking, running) coordination patterns. Both patterns are stable attractors; it is difficult to shift away from them for more than short periods of time.

Skilled performance, which develops over time, has elements of both stability (as evidenced from reduced variability) and flexibility (as evidenced by the ability to recover from a perturbation). These attractor states provide the basis from which novel motor performance can emerge. However, children with autism have difficulty achieving stable attractor states upon which they can build new skills and scaffold to a gain or permanent change in abilities.

Practitioners can interpret the process of intervention as change between or among stable attractor states, preferably from a less to more adaptive movement pattern. While understanding the nature of stablity is important, so is understanding the complementary nature of change. One of the hallmarks of change is variablitiy. Prior to the use of an ecological perspective, researchers and practitioners considered variablitiy to be intrinsic to movement impairment, something that decreased with increased recovery, practice, or intervention. This created the problematic situation of statistical analysis. Often, both inter and intra-individual variablity made statistical inference difficult, as wide standard deviation bands masked any age-related differences that may exist. However, researchers using an ecological perspective have embraced the study of variablity, by examining the dynamic stablity of movements over varying timescales (29). That is to say, the structure of variablity became meaningful and more than just a marker of improving (or changing) skill. Researchers examining different types of motor impairment have successfully examined structure in variablity to understand both the nature of impairment and the success of intervention (21).

Multileveled, multi-determined, and interactive processes lead to motor control and coordination. Because movement results from a self-organizing, non-linear series of emergent attractor states, no one structure or level can be held accountable for the movements seen any children, typically developing or with ASD (27). Each level is independent while at the same time, interdependent, so that small changes in one level may result in large changes at another level. In relation to movement impairment in children with ASD, this suggests that small changes such as modified sensory perceptual input, task complexity, or muscular stiffness may result in larger behavioral shifts. Further, it implicates the transactional nature of perception, cognition, and action in emergent behavior. That is, not only does one system influence others, it is, in turn, changed by the resultant emergent behavior.

Previous research on motor deficits in individuals with ASD

The next step in using an ecological perspective to examine individuals with ASD involves reviewing what we know about motor impairment in this population, regardless of the theoretical perspective used to frame this knowledge. This will help to identify which individual characteristics appear to be most influential, and where in the process of perception, cognition, and action coupling individuals with ASD are most impaired. This information was derived through an extensive literature review using various search engines such as Pubmed and Psychinfo.

Children with ASD typically show difficulty with motor skills (praxis), especially if the task is novel. These children typically have difficulty with timing, sequencing, initiation, and transitioning (14) as well as force control (30). We have focused on two specific bodies of literature examining motor deficits that suggest that the use of an ecological perspective may be beneficial to the study of ASD. These are motor imitation and anticipatory deficits.

Motor imitation abilities

Children with autism have deficits in motor imitation, a skill requiring interaction among perception, cognition, and action. To successfully imitate a movement, one must perceive (generally through visual and auditory systems) the actions of another person, interpret that movement, develop a strategy for performing the action, cognitively transform the action into an individual body scale and referenced axes of rotation, and then move in one's own immediate environment. During the actual motor output of imitation efforts, the child's system must gain intact feedback from visual, auditory, and proprioceptive input "real time" while performing the action to self-adjust and refine the imitation effort. Literature findings point to two different presentations of problems in motor imitation in which children with ASD are delayed or are deviant in the development of imitation skills which may predict play and language deficits (17): deficits in action production (delayed) or in action perception (deviant).

Children with ASD have a more difficult time with non-object oriented (ie: body movement) imitation than they have with object oriented imitation compared to typically developing children (16,17). Difficulty with body movement imitation appears early in development and extends through at least adolescence (31). In a study evaluating imitation in children with low and high functioning autism, regardless level of functioning, all children eventually achieved some resemblance of imitation. However, both groups of children required more effort in trial number to attempt to imitate 24 gestures and demonstrated errors in targeting and position accuracy in final imitation stance compared to children developing typically and those with learning disabilities (16). Such findings suggest challenges in action production may underlie motor impairments as well as be influenced by perception and cognition (4).

Children with autism also have difficulty with imitation of object oriented imitation. One study found 8-year-old to 12-year-old children with autism, were less successful with object oriented imitation than body movement orientation and suggested results represent a deviance in developmental pattern of motor imitation. Mostofsky et al. (3) found that children with autism have a more difficult time with object oriented imitation than with non-object oriented imitation.

Two possible explanations for the delayed or deveient differences exist. First, the findings may represent a developmental transition in motor imitation impairments, with younger children initially doing more poorly in body movement imitation becoming older school aged children who then have difficulty with object use perception affecting object imitation. In other words, initial motor imitation issues are related to action production, and build across development to become more related to perception action deficits. Secondly, the variability in findings may reflect the wide range of phenotypes of children on the spectrum of autism. Some children may display delayed development of action production systems (body imitation is harder than object imitation) while other children may have a different pathology contributing to an actual difference in action perception systems (when object imitation is harder than body imitation). In other words, it may be possible that some children have action production as a primary impairment (body movement group) such as poor body awareness affecting imitation of body movements. Primary impairments in feedback systems during motor action may influence this group. Meanwhile, other clusters of children have action perception (object oriented) related impairments, with deficits in feed forward systems influencing motor action. Longitudinal studies following children from pre-school through adolescents may help advance explanation of motor imitation deficits in autism. Studies considering performance on perceptual tasks using fMRI emerging in the literature suggest a role for perceptual differences to affect motor outcomes. The link may be in the impact of perception and action upon the child's ability to anticipate, gather information, and respond accordinatly during a daily activity.

Perception-action and anticipation: Influences on motor abilities

Central nervous system differences in perceptual skills and anticipatory function influence motor performance in healthy, typically developing sample groups. Typically developing children have brain activity as well as different ectodermal and eye fixation motor responses with the visual presentation of novel stimuli or novel targets in an activity (32,33). Children with autism and poor motor skills have poor ability to attend and orient to peripheral attention cues compared to children with autism who do not have poor motor skills and with typically developing peers (12). Attention to task with and without environmental distractions empowers an individual with the ability to interpret environmental cues and adeptly select appropriate motor responses for successful engagement in the environment. In this fashion, anticipatory function occurs with the environmental interpretation of known cues with flexibility regardless environmental distractions or novel stimuli. Processing of "in view" and "distractor" tasks may have common neurological pathways (34). Thus, in the example of the child transitioning between train play and a family meal may yield poor transition and outcome as a result of the child's difficulty in anticipating the adult command, and resultant deviation and processing and planning a congruent motor and behavioral response. Because children with autism have deficits in anticipation skills, it may be possible that their decreased attention orienting and sensory processing skills negatively affect anticipatory during novel tasks or in novel environments. This reduced capacity of anticipatory guidance, in turn, may yield motor control problems.

Evidence in both sensory and motor-based findings exists to support central nervous system differences in children with autism during tasks requiring anticipatory skill. Brain activity responses differ in children with autism compared to age matched peers with the presentation of an unprompted auditory stimulus during non-task specific time periods (9,35, 36). Processing unfamiliar verbal information in context is difficult for children with autism

(9). Functionally, a child with autism's difficulty with motor actions upon verbal command may reflect these differences in processing auditory stimulus both with and without task specificity. Further support for decreased anticipation skills and central nervous system functioning is found in visual stimulus processing.

Visual perceptual processing in children with autism demonstrates differences in central nervous system functioning lending to decreased integrity in stimulus processing and response with increasing stimulus complexity (37). In addition, decreased visual perceptual processing may impact/be impacted by decreased integrity of a neurological observation-execution matching system (38). Results from a motor task, lifting of a bimanual load, suggest further anticipatory deficits with respect to activation of muscle fiber contraction (30). Overall, it is possible that anticipatory deficits contribute to the establishment and integrity of gross motor plans by children on the autistic spectrum, thus lending to their presentation of motor impairments on standardized assessment tools.

Discussion

There are many ways in which researchers studying ASD can used these and other principles of an ecological perspective to guide both design and interpretation of empirical research. We would like to offer both specific ideas and general thoughts as starting points for such a research agenda.

Motor imitation issues: non-linear phase shifts. Impairment in motor imitation may take a non-linear trajectory through development: during early childhood, children with autism may have issues with non-object oriented motor imitation and this shifts to an impairment in object oriented motor imitation as children get older. Such developmental, non-linear shifts are suggestive of complex systems. Initially, relatively stable attractor states exist for these systems. Over time, one or several critical constraints change or are scaled up or down through the process of development. Once a critical level of this constraint is reached, the system responds first by increasing the amount of variability present, and then by restructuring around a new attractor state (39).

Do the changes from non-object oriented to object oriented impairments in motor imitation represent a non-linear phase shift? One could examine this by following a group of children with and without ASD over a period of several years. Researchers would provide both groups with body and object oriented motor imitation tasks during separate testing sessions. Individuals' responses to motor imitations could be tracked on a session-to-session basis and analyzed for the presence of attractor states. This would continue for a predetermined number of trials and testing sessions. Based on our earlier discussion of motor imitation impairment, we predict one of two potential outcomes may exist. In one, no phase shift occurs. The children with ASD do not transition from non-object to object orientation deficits (or do not initially show non-object impairment, which would suggest that specific phenotypes within individuals with ASD exist. Alternatively, a phase shift does occur. At this point, researchers would examine concurrent developmental changes in perception, cognition, and action to see if associations can be found between specific individual constraints and motor imitation impairment.

Anticipatory deficits: Unpacking perception, cognition, and action. Using a series of empirical studies, researchers could begin to unpack the influences of perception, cognition, and action and their influences on anticipatory deficits with this population. One way researchers can achieve this is through the manipulation of task demands in terms of specific coupling requirement (perception-cognition, cognition-action). For example, one could explore the role of perception-cognition coupling using a simple motor task that requires no anticipation and little movement, such as a reaction time task. Initial trials would involve the determination of a stable attractor state for a given sensory. To determine the role of perception, researchers could systematically alter different types and amounts of sensory stimuli. For example, the color of the light could change, or researchers could provide an auditory stimulus. Differences seen in reaction time would represent differences in perception-cognition coupling. In order to increase anticipatory levels, researchers could also vary conditions to increase complexity and cognitive requirements while keeping sensory input constant. Differences should provide insight into the relative roles of perception and cognition in a simple RT task. Similarly, researchers could perform a series of studies to examine the role of anticipation in cognitive-action coupling. Initially, sensory stimuli must remain constant throughout the task, and motor response must be relatively complex.

In order to examine the role that anticipation plays in performance, researchers can manipulate temporal coordination with or without adding sensory stimuli. In typically developing populations, stable attractor states emerge as individuals anticipate spatial and temporal requirements of the task; the time course of this stability could be compared to that of the population with ASD. Further, once stable attractor states emerge, researchers can suddenly apply perturbations to examine the role of anticipation in producing initial stable attractors as well as return to stability.

One important consideration when examining anticipatory responses in individuals with ASD is the role of context or environment. Any efforts to maintain ecological validity within the context of an experiment should result in a better representation of functional deficit. For example, asking a participant to match a metronome beat by tapping his or her finger is a highly controlled, yet artificial task. Participants with ASD may respond in two ways: they may perform better than in a more natural environmental context because of reduced sensory stimuli and motor action. The possibility exists that they may perform worse than in more natural context as well, because they may not prescribe any meaning to a novel task as described by the researcher (due to issues with social communication). Keeping that in mind, researchers should attempt to make tasks play-based, and try to replicate 'typical' environmental settings.

Conclusion

Based on an ecological perspective, we suggest four new directions for research to explore the skills and challenges of children and adults with ASD. First, researchers should pay greater attention to the interrelated aspect of multiple systems. This can benefit study of ASD by bringing together pieces of the puzzle (perception, cognition, action) generally observed in isolation of others. Such multi-layered research paradigms may enable new areas of study, and offer different explanations for previously observed phenomena. From co-actional, dynamic research, theoretically based interventions can be generated and tested, and both quantitatively and qualitatively compared to predicted results. Second, evolution of new paradigms or alterations of existing paradigms are required to gain further insight into the cognition, perception, action challenges of children with autism. In this manner, a researcher can examine the effect of perceptual complexity as the child moves from environments with low to high perceptual information. Third, current research in autism identifies variability in performance as a problem in autism. Thus, further research, embracing the sheer nature of variability in performance; occur in order to establish the nature and influence of variability upon change across developmental and chronological time. Fourth, children with autism appear to present with anticipatory deficits amidst the dynamic interaction of cognition, perception, and action, which would benefit from further research attention.

References

[1] American Psychological Association. Diagnostic and statistical manual of mental disorders, 5th ed. Washington, DC: APA, 2000.

[2] World Health Organization. International classifications of diseases (ICD-10). Chapter 5: Disorders of psychological development (F80-F89). Retrieved on-line (October 15, 2008). www.who.int/classifications /apps/icd/icd10online/2007

[3] Mostofsky SH, Dubey P, Jerath VK, Jansiewicz EM, Goldberg MC, Denckla MB. Developmental dyspraxia is not limited to imitation in children with autism spectrum disorders. J. Int. Neuropsych. Soc. 2006;12(3):314-26.

[4] Dewey D, Cantell M, Crawford SG. Motor and gestural performance in children with autism spectrum disorders, developmental coordination disorder, and/or attention deficit hyperactivity disorder. J. of Int. Neuropsych. Soc. 2007;13(2):246-56

[5] Gidley Larson JC, Bastian AJ, Donchin O, Shadmehr R, Mostofsky, SH. Acquisition of internal models of motor tasks in children with autism. Brain. 2008;131(Pt 11):2894-903.

[6] Huebner RA. Autism: A sensorimotor approach to management. Gaithersburg, MD: Aspen, 2001.

[7] Schaff RC, Miller LC. Occupational therapy using a sensory integrative approach for children with developmental disabilities. Ment. Retard. Dev. Disabil. Res. Rev. 2005;11:142-8.

[8] Williams DL, Goldstein G, Minshew, NJ. Neuropsychologic functioning in children with autism: further evidence for disordered complex information-processing. Child. Neuropsychol. 2006;12(4-5):279-98.

[9] Lopez B, Leekam S. Do children with autism fail to process information in context? J. Child Psychol. Psychiatry. 2003;44(2):285-300.

[10] Caron MJ, Mottron L, Berthiaume C, Dawson M. Cognitive mechanisms,specificity and neural underpinnings of visuospatial peaks in autism. Brain. 2006;129(Pt 7):1789-802.

[11] Gastab HZ, Strauss MS, Minshew NJ Do individuals with autism process categories differently? The effect of typicality and development. Child Dev. 2006;77(6):1717-29.

[12] Renner P, Grofer Klinger L, Klinger MR Exogenous and endogenous attention orienting in autism spectrum disorders. Child Neuropsychol. 2006;12(4-5):361-82.

[13] Martineua J, Schmitz C, Assaiante C, Blanc R, Barthelemy C. Impairment of a cortical event-related desynchronisation during a bimanual load lifting task in children with autistic disorder. Neurosci. Lett. 2004;367:298-303.

[14] Miller-Kuhaneck H. Autism: A comprehensive occupational therapy approach. Bethesda, MD: AOTA Press, 2004.

[15] Rinehart N, Bellgrove M, Tonge B, Brereton A, Howells-Rankin D, Bradshaw JL. An examination of movement kinematics in young people with high functioning autism and asperger's disorder: further evidence for a motor planning deficit. J. Autism Dev. Disord. 2006;36:757-67.

[16] Vanvuchelen M, Roeyers H, De Weerdt W. Nature of motor imitation problems in school-aged males with autism: how congruent are the error types? Dev. Med. Child Neurol. 2007;49(1):6-12.

[17] Stone WL, Ousley OY, & Littleford CD. Motor imitation in young children with autism: What's the object? J. Abnorm. Child Psychol. 1997;25(6):475-85.

[18] Adolph KE, Vereijken B, Shrout PE. What changes in infant walking and why. Child Dev. 2003;74:475-97.

[19] Dingwell JB, Cusumano JP, Sternad D, Cavanagh PR. Slower speeds in patients with diabetic neuropathy lead to improved local dynamic stability of continuous overground walking. J. Biomech. 2000;33:1269-77.

[20] Getchell N, McMenamin S, Whitall J. Dual motor task coordination in children with and without learning disabilities. Adapt. Phys. Activ. Q. 2005;22:21-38.

[21] Buzzi UH, Ulrich BD. Dynamic stability of gait cycles as a function of speed and system constraints. Motor Control. 2004;8(3):241-54.

[22] Whitall J, Getchell N, McMenamin S, Horn C, Wilms-Floet A, Clark J. Perception-action coupling in children with and without DCD: Frequency locking between task relevant auditory signals and motor responses in a dual motor task. Child Care Health Dev. 2006;32:679- 92

[23] Sternad D. Debates in dynamics: A dynamic systems perspective to perception and action. Hum. Movement Sci. 2000;19:407-23.

[24] Thelen E. Grounded in the world: Developmental origins of the embodied mind. Infancy. 2000;1:3-28.

[25] Kelso JAS, Engstrøm DA. The complementary nature. Cambridge, MA: MIT Press, 2006.

[26] Clarke D, Crossland H. Action systems: An introduction to the analysis of complex behaviour. London: Methuen,1985.

[27] Newell K. Physical constraints to development of motor skills. In: Thomas J, ed. Motor development during childhood and adolescence. Minneapolis, MN: Burgess,1984.

[28] Klin A, Jones W, Schulz R, Volkmar F. The enactive mind, or from actions to cognition: lessons from autism. Phil. Trans. R. Soc. Lond. B. 2003;358:345-60.

[29] Deutsch KM, Newell KM. Noise, variability, and the development of children's perceptual-motor skills. Dev. Rev. 2005;25:155-80.

[30] Schmitz C, Martineau J, Barthelemy C, Assainte C. Motor control and children with autism: deficit in anticipatory function? Neurosci. Lett. 2003;348:17-20.

[31] Freitag CM, Kleser C, Gontard A. Imitation and language abilities in adolescents with Autism Spectrum Disorder without language delay. Eur. Child Adolesc. Psychiatry. 2006;15(5):282.

[32] Van Engeland H, Roelofs J, Verbaten M, Slangen J. Abnormal electrodermal reactivity to novel visual stimuli in autistic children. Psychiatry Res. 1991;38(1):27-38.

[33] Clark V, Fannon S, Lai S, Benson R, Bauer L. Responses to rare visual target and distractor stimuli using event related fMRI. J. Neurophysiol. 2000;83:3133-9.

[34] Bledowski C, Prvulovic D, Goebel R, Zanella F, Linden D. Attentional systems in target and distractor processing: a combined ERP and fMRI study. Neuroimage. 2004;22:530-40.

[35] Gomot M, Bernard F, Davis M, Belmonte M, Ashwin C, Bullmore E, Baron-Cohen S. Change detection in children with autism: an auditory event related fMRI study. NeuroImage. 2006;29:475-84.

[36] Minshew NJ, Williams DL. The new neurobiology of autism: Cortex, connectivity and neuronal organization. Arch. Neurol. 2007;64:945-50.

[37] Bertone A, Motron L, Jelenic P, Faubert J. Enhanced and diminished visual spatial information processing in autism depends on stimulus complexity. Brain. 2005;128:2430-41.

[38] Lepage JF, Theoret H. EEG evidence for the presence of an action observation-execution matching system in children. Eur. J. Neurosci. 2006;23(9):2505-10.

[39] Diedrich FJ, Warren WH. Why change gaits? Dynamics of the walk-run transition. J. Exp. Psychol. Hum. Percept. Perform. 1995;21:183-202.

In: Understanding Autism Spectrum Disorder
Editors: Ditza A Zachor and Joav Merrick

ISBN: 978-1-62081-353-9

Chapter 2

It takes a village: Redefining kin, extended family, and other social networks in the treatment of childhood autism

Jennifer Hillman [*] ***and Elon Gruber***
The Pennsylvania State University, Berks College,
Applied Psychology Program, Pennsylvania, US

Abstract

Epidemiological findings suggest that with 1 in 166 children diagnosed with an autism spectrum disorder each year, 1 in 46 families also are affected. Unique stressors of autism upon families typically include social isolation and financial burden. The need to provide the minimum treatment recommended by the Surgeon General of the United States of nearly 40 hours a week of specialized therapy, coupled with typically disruptive behavioral symptoms and concomitant medical problems, adds additional challenges for family members, particularly for working mothers. The presence of mental illness and family dysfunction can also impair the ability of family members to provide a diagnosed child with appropriate treatment. Parents of autistic children are more likely to experience depression, anxiety, and marital distress than parents of both typical children and those with mental retardation. Although family therapy remains an essential mode of treatment for nuclear families, it is recommended that the social network of the family be expanded significantly to include grandparents, other extended family, neighbors, church and other community groups, and formal and informal support groups with significant benefit for both the identified child and the affected family. For example, the role of active grandparent can be expanded to include geographically distant and foster grandparents. In response to social isolation, the use of technology, including the internet, will be discussed as a unique mode of social and informational support. Case examples will illustrate the benefits of such an expanded approach in family based treatment.

---

[*] Correspondence: Dr. Jennifer Hillman, Professor of Psychology, The Pennsylvania State University, Berks College, Tulpehocken Rd, PO Box 7009, Reading, PA 19610, USA. E-mail: JHillman@psu.edu.

Introduction

Although some experts are in disagreement about whether or not the incidence of autism has reached epidemic proportions, most agree with recent reports that indicate 1 out of 166 children in the United States suffer from an autism spectrum disorder (1). Related statistics suggest that 1 out of 46 families are directly affected. As defined by the Diagnostic and Statistical Manual of Mental Disorders (2), autism is a pervasive developmental disorder in which a child presents with significant impairment or delays in both verbal and non-verbal communication, particularly in relation to social interaction, and stereotypical, repetitive, and apparently non-functional behaviors, interests, and activities. Pretend or imaginative play is typically absent. Bizarre or repetitive physical movements (e.g., hand flapping), lack of eye contact, a desire for adherence to routines, abnormal posturing, and rage or self-injurious behaviors also may be present.

To complicate matters further, many children with autism present with significant, concomitant medical problems including seizures, gastrointestinal problems (e.g., ulcerative colitis; chronic constipation or diarrhea), sleep disturbances, food allergies or sensitivities, sensory-motor disturbances (e.g., sensitivity to certain sounds; poor gross and fine motor coordination), feeding disorders (i.e., inability or unwillingness to eat), chronic ear or other infections, and hypotonia (i.e., muscle weakness) among others (3). For every girl who is diagnosed with autism, four or five more boys receive the diagnosis. For purposes of simplicity in this chapter, the term "autism" will be used broadly to represent both autism and Pervasive Developmental Disorder Not Otherwise Specified (PDD-NOS), which is sometimes controversially referred to as "high-functioning" autism. The etiology or cause of autism also remains unclear. Overall, it is important to note that autism, as a developmental disorder, appears multi-faceted and presents itself uniquely among each affected child and family.

Standard approaches to treatment

According to the Surgeon General's Office of the United States, the recommended form of treatment for childhood autism is 30-40 hours of an intensive, one-on-one behaviorally based treatment known as Applied Behavioral Analysis (ABA; (4)). ABA is derived from now classic research conducted by Lovaas (5), in which children with autism who engaged in the recommended hours of discrete trial learning daily for at least two years significantly raised their IQ scores and were able to function in a typical, versus special education, first grade classroom. Additional, emergent variants of this seminal treatment include ABA for Verbal Behavioral Model and Natural Environment Training, in which children with autism are helped specifically to communicate verbally and develop appropriate behaviors in more naturalistic and community-based settings (3). Significant limitations of ABA and its modern options include a staggering annual cost of $25,000-$40,000 U.S. with only limited reimbursement from most insurance plans, limited numbers of trained and available staff, and a lack of long-term outcome research (6). Also unfortunately, although both classic and more modern ABA programs require parents to be involved in the delivery of treatment, these approaches focus exclusively upon the identified patient; family therapy is not required or even formally recommended.

Within the last decade, additional psychologically-based treatments for autism have been developed that expand the role of parents in their child's treatment. Some of these treatment approaches are more controversial than others, and the majority offer limited empirical support despite positive anecdotal reports from parents and teachers. One promising approach to treatment is Relationship Development Intervention (RDI), in which parents must complete intensive training and psychoeducation about autism, as well as typical cognitive and social development, before they can begin to work with their own affected child as a "guide" or "coach." Parents are taught to regain their "expert status" as parent of their own child and family. A recently published empirical study (7) indicates that all 16 children diagnosed with autism on the Autism Diagnostic Observation Schedule (ADOS), a standardized and generally well-respected diagnostic measure, who were treated with RDI for at least two and a half years no longer qualified for a formal diagnosis of autism via post treatment assessment with the ADOS. Additional child gains were reported in cognitive flexibility as well as regular versus special educational placement. Although the study itself suffers from a lack of a formal comparison group, its initial findings suggest that additional controlled studies should be conducted and RDI as a treatment model should be explored.

RDI places significant emphasis upon helping parents address their own mental health needs (e.g., make time for yourself; see a therapist if you feel depressed), reduce overall levels of stress for all family members (e.g., spend special time alone with neurotypical siblings), and increase their sense of hope or vision for a positive future. Potential problems or barriers to the delivery of RDI among families affected by autism, however, include the high cost (e.g., thousands of dollars a year) and the need to hire a private, uniquely certified RDI consultant. As with ABA, in many geographic areas the demand for qualified consultants and therapists significantly outweighs the number available. Other impediments for parents seeking to adopt RDI include difficulties in obtaining insurance reimbursement, a general lack of acceptance in public schools, and a need for video equipment and specialized computer access available only through the RDI treatment center. Despite these limitations, RDI is one of the few approaches to the treatment of autism that demands both familial involvement and assessment. In accord with general principles of family therapy, in RDI the family unit itself is considered the cornerstone of healing. Family therapists can work within this context as significant agents of family health and change.

Role of child's condition on the family

Parents of a child with a disability must confront the unique stressors introduced by the disability, which are intensified by severity of the condition. Specifically, 16% of parents whose child's disability (defined in a recent survey to include children with autism who have difficulties with activities of daily living) was categorized as mild to moderate reported that their child's health was their chief source of daily stress, as compared to 38% of parents whose child's disability was classified as severe to very severe (8). Additionally, parents' personal expectations for themselves concerning how involved they should be in providing assistance for their child also were affected by the severity of the disability. Nearly four in five of those with a child with a severe disability felt dissatisfied by the assistance that they were providing for their child as compared to approximately one in two parents whose child's disability was classified as mild to moderate (8). Parental stress appears to vary with the type of problems exhibited by children with autism. Baker et al. (9) reported that a disabled child's behavioral difficulties are a better predictor of stress for parents than the child's developmental delay. Furthermore, specific behavioral problems (e.g., aggressive behaviors) are more highly associated with elevated levels of stress for parents than adaptive behaviors for not only children, but adolescents with autism (10).

The majority of studies to date have focused on the association between the DSM characteristics of autism and increasing levels of stress for mothers, particularly in relation to repetitious, atypical behaviors and sleep deprivation (11). Also of importance, however, are the potentially differing, individual positions of both the mother and father regarding their autistic child's most problematic and stressful behaviors. Davis and Carter (12) found that mothers were most concerned with the child's deficient self-regulation abilities (e.g., eating), whereas fathers were more affected by bizarre, nonfunctional behaviors (e.g., hand flapping), which can elicit disapproving attention from others, and poor communication skills. Related studies indicate that mothers are apprehensive about their children's capability to function independently, their future wellbeing, and the community's perception and acceptance of their children (13), whereas fathers are more concerned about finances and interference with planning events that involve the family (14). It is recommended here that further exploration should include both parents' perceptions of individual sources of stress.

The relationship among employment, finances and cost of care

Most parents of a child with autism also have to adapt to modifications in employment, which typically involve a constriction of options and decrease in income. Employment is most influenced by a reduction in the amount of hours worked, which appears to be profoundly impacted by the severity of the child's disability. For example, one-third of Canadian mothers reported working fewer hours to provide care for their disabled child. Additionally, nearly 20% reported that they turned down a promotion, while another 21% terminated employment (8). Primarily, mothers appear most affected by employment alterations. A U.S. survey found that 84% of mothers with disabled children were not in paid employment compared with 39% of mothers with non disabled children (15).

Additional findings suggest that significantly more single mothers and grandmothers assume care for a disabled child and exit the workforce to encounter additional financial strain (16). These changes have important financial implications that can increase stress for families. In fact, parents who have a child with a severe disability were three time more likely to indicate that they have experienced financial strain or difficulties within the last year, mainly attributed to the cost of care (8). Overall, these research findings suggest that women mainly encounter the burden of being a fulltime caregiver, and often are forced to discontinue working to assume this position, even though maintaining employment outside of the home is associated with increased ratings of happiness for both mothers and fathers (17) and a greater likelihood of providing the recommended, costly care for their autistic child.

Impact upon siblings

Siblings frequently offer emotional, social and practical support for one another. However, when a sibling has a disability, the support may expand beyond what is characteristically expected of the relationship. Although little has been published about the bond that people with autism have with their siblings, Orsmond and Seltzer (18) reported that siblings of individuals with Down Syndrome were more hopeful about their sibling's future and had a more intimate relationship with their brother and sister as compared to those who had a sibling with autism. The authors propose that these differences may be due to the presence of certain "strange" or non-functional behaviors typically exhibited by people with autism, or the autistic sibling's inability to engage in social interaction. Siblings of autistic children also may assume the role of caregiver for their brother or sister with autism once their parents can no longer fulfill the position, and they may confront more challenges than those with a sibling with Down syndrome because of the lack of emotional closeness and behavioral support (18).

Individuals with a disabled sibling report struggles with social isolation, limited family contact, adjustment problems, lower self esteem and communication difficulties (e.g., (19)). Anecdotal as well as documented accounts exist of siblings being seriously injured by an autistic sibling. The brothers and sisters of autistic children also appear likely to experience embarrassment, confusion, and fear in relation to their sibling's inappropriate or atypical behavior, as well as resentment related to what may be perceived as an unfair distribution of the parents' time and financial resources (3,6). It does appear helpful to the non-disabled sibling to be immediately and sufficiently informed about their sibling's diagnosis, as communicating that information appears to relate to how optimistically these individuals consider their siblings' disability to have a more positive versus negative impact upon their lives (20).

Unique marital stressors

The multiple stressors related to a change in marital dynamics when a couple has children can be intensified if one of the children has a disability-- particularly that of autism. The rates of marriage are lower and the incidence of divorce is higher for parents of disabled children (21). Moreover, marital conflicts lead to divorce in more than three of four marriages with disabled children (8). Parents who have a child with a severe disability were twice as likely to report marital problems (43%) attributed to the disability as compared to parents with a child whose disability was classified as mild to moderate (8). The most frequently reported problems were stress or depression (85%), and disagreements or arguments (84%) directly related to their child's condition. Additional findings indicate that parents with a child suffering from autism report greater levels of stress than parents with a child diagnosed with Down Syndrome, cerebral palsy (22), and mental retardation (23). A related study (24) found that parents of a child with autism experience dissatisfaction with domains such as time spent together, child rearing (e.g., discipline), and sexual intimacy. Conversely, strategies such as active problem-solving and affectively based communication were associated with strengths within the family, and may operate as a barrier for stress.

The impact upon grandparents

Grandparenthood is portrayed as an enjoyable and appreciated transition, which allows for a reconnection with the past. However, for grandparents with a disabled child, many of these grandparents may go through a period of mourning, during which they grieve for the loss of the grandchild and the relationship they expected to have, and then begin to adapt to their new role (25). This period of adjustment may be impeded if the grandparents receive inadequate information about the grandchild's diagnosis. Specifically, a lack of knowledge concerning the grandchild's disability and related symptoms appears to contribute to not only a state of role confusion among grandparents with autism (26), but also fear, guilt and potential conflict with parents. A qualitative study of biological grandparents' responses to their relationship with an autistic child (26) revealed three primary areas of concern. These included remaining protective towards their adult child and grandchild, searching for meaning in relation to the diagnosis of autism, and working to maintain family relations. The majority of these grandparents also expressed a clear need for social support in relation to stressors of autism in their family.

Grandparental support, particularly from the grandmother, has been demonstrated to be beneficial for not only young mothers, but also for children whose parents are divorced (27). Often grandparents of non-disabled children provide complimentary childcare for parents who are employed full time. Grandparents frequently provide childcare for parents who work, particularly on the weekends or in the evenings, or who have a child enrolled in a part-time pre-school program (28). As noted previously, some grandparents help provide care for an autistic grandchild so that their adult daughter can work. The necessity for childcare may lessen as neurotypical children become teenagers; but for families with an autistic child, childcare concerns may persist and become even more complex (3, 28).

The impact of grandparents upon the family

Most of the literature concerning grandparents and a grandchild's disability has focused upon the mothers' perception of the emotional experience. Research indicates that there is a hierarchy of perceived support, with maternal grandmothers receiving the highest ratings and reports of satisfaction from both mothers and fathers (25), primarily because they are credited as the most essential figures in providing emotional support to the mother (30). Close mother-daughter relationships have been associated with reduced paternal stress, however, less emotionally involved relationships between the mother and daughter-in-law have been shown to produce an elevated level of stress for mothers of disabled children (31). Maternal grandparents appear to provide more frequent support than paternal grandparents, although fathers report reduced stress levels when both maternal and paternal grandparents have involvement (31).

Grandparental support, which may include both practical (e.g., caregiving for respite care and work related activities; advocacy) and emotionally supportive contributions (e.g., listening; providing non-judgmental advice) are typically appreciated by parents (30). Additional reports of formal and informal support include monetary assistance, transportation, help with medical appointments and behavioral problems, assistance with household chores, regular visits, and service as paraprofessionals (29). Grandparents may provide differing degrees of involvement and assistance based on various factors, although the importance of support appears less reliant upon geographical distance than upon emotional availability (32).

Some reasons for modest grandparental involvement include health conditions, perception of burden, resentment resulting from a loss of earned income (33), perceived loss of personal freedom (27), and previous conflicts or poor relationship with adult children (34). Despite these potential barriers, research from grandparents of children with developmental disabilities suggests that a stronger bond or relationship between grandparents themselves can result from increased involvement (35). Another important consideration is that the more grandparents are involved in open communication with parents regarding their grandchild's diagnosis of autism and related treatment, the more likely they are to provide the types of support consistent with the parents' needs (3).

Cultural and individual differences in grandparenting

Currently, there are no empirical studies involving the racial or cultural influences among grandparents of children with autism, however, there are a few available studies regarding African-American (36), Latino (37) and Panamanian (38) grandparents of children with disabilities. Many African-American and Latino families place considerable emphasis on unity within the family, and endorse expectations of emotional and instrumental support among all generations (39). Various studies indicate that both Latino (37) and African-American custodial grandparents of children with developmental disabilities (36) are at significant risk for depressive symptoms. For many of these grandparents, being single, not working outside of the home, and having limited education were associated with greater symptomology (36). It is crucial to examine additional, potential differences among grandparents of children with autism, including geographic location, socioeconomic status, health status, household composition, caregiver status, and employment, which may be linked with culture and ethnicity.

Recommendations for expansion of the kin network

As noted, an actively engaged grandparent can provide significant benefits to the entire family, as well as the identified child, affected by autism. The following section is designed to offer specific recommendations to increase grandparental involvement, and also to offer alternative means to expand the family's kin network if biological grandparents are not available or amenable. For example, grandparents should be one of the primary candidates to receive information about autism during the child's initial assessment of autism and subsequent intervention (29). Providing grandparents with related social supports also appears important. Although few formal evaluations of existing support groups (e.g., the Autism Society of America's Generations Club) appear in the literature, the reports available do suggest that grandparents consider these an encouraging experience, as they value the opportunity to become better educated, engage in investigative group activities, and share experiences with others who appreciate and recognize their difficulties (40).

For grandparents who are at a geographic distance or who may have health impairments, the use of technology such as the internet, including e-mail and web cam systems (e.g., Skype), can allow previously unavailable or uninvolved grandparents to become significantly involved in their grandchild or adult child's struggle and treatment of autism. Even at a distance, grandparents can be encouraged to act as advocates, either exclusively on the grandchild's behalf or for the entire family. Many families appear unaware of various tax deductions related to medical treatments and special education regulations related to autism. Although empirical research is needed to assess the outcome of such internet-based grandparental involvement, anecdotal reports suggest that any type of support is beneficial to family members affected by autism.

The role of foster grandparent also needs to be examined as a potential source of support for families with autistic children (3, 29). Foster grandparents can be sought to develop special relationships and supports among parents and neurotypical siblings as well as the identified child with autism. Both formal and informal means can be used to engage a middle-aged or older adult in this capacity. Formal means can include an expansion of existing, community-based foster grandparent programs or via the establishment of new programs with centers of higher education that will provide foster candidates with education and even some monetary support. Informal and sometimes necessarily more creative means can include seeking out an older adult through a local senior center, retirement home, or local neighborhood or religious community. Anecdotal reports suggest that many older adults who are approached with such a request are flattered and seek to find out more information. Parents also should be directed to be as straightforward and open as possible with the potential foster grandparent regarding their and their child's specific needs and wants for support, and to develop mutually acceptable expectations for participation in specific activities and the types and frequency of interaction. Clinical experience of the first author also suggests that older adults who may not have young or school age grandchildren of their own, or who are disappointed that they have limited involvement with their own grandchildren due to geographic constraints or other factors, are typically good candidates.

Similarly, neighbors, local religious groups, and other informal support groups can provide extended kin support. For example, one Autism Society of America local chapter organized a series of social outings and parties for families, particularly around holidays. Sample activities included the renting of a local movie theater for a preview of a new children's movie, free hay rides during a harvest festival, an independence day picnic at a reserved park pavilion, etc. The plan behind these events was to literally find a "safe place" for parents, siblings, and their children with autism to play and spend time together, without having to worry about explaining their child's behavior to others. Additional recreational and support groups were created specifically for the neurotypical siblings. Of course, this chapter included public awareness and education as other programming, but for a few hours each month, families spend time together and meet with other families with similar needs and issues. Therapists also can encourage parents to form their own informal support groups. On-line chat and support groups can provide outstanding support for parents and family members who may be socially isolated due to long work hours, lack of respite care, or their child's severe behavioral problems, as well as those who are geographically distant from established centers of care (e.g., those in rural areas.)

Case examples

The following case examples are offered to demonstrate some of the issues that family therapists may encounter in work with a family affected by autism, as well as some options for expanding those families' kin and social networks. Please note that these case examples are meant for illustrative purposes, and that they do not represent all families' experiences. Every family affected by autism is unique, and must be assessed and treated as such.

Sasha was an 8 year-old girl diagnosed with autism. Her family consisted of her biological mother, Lorraine, who was divorced, and a 13 year-old sister, Patty. Sasha's biological father moved to another state and had no real contact with either of his daughters. Lorraine believed she was doing well with her daughters and Sasha's care. Sasha attended a special education program at her local school, and Lorraine began receiving disturbing reports from the teachers indicating that Sasha began using foul language and acting aggressively with children who previously were her friends. After a few meetings with the school district, it was determined that Sasha's older sister, Patty, had been telling Sasha to go to school and say or do certain things (e.g., "If you don't like your homework, tell your teacher, 'Kiss my ass,' and hit (your friend) in the arm really hard to show them how much you like them.") Lorraine was shocked at her eldest daughter's behavior, and immediately called a family therapist for help.

Upon further exploration, the family therapist found out that Patty was extremely angry and upset in response to what she perceived as a significant and unnecessary drain upon their family's resources for Sasha's special schooling, ABA treatment, and medical bills. Patty explained that for a few years, "I just thought Sasha would get better, and there would finally be some time and money for me." Patty said that "I just lost it when I asked Mom for the last time to take me to my friend's house, and she said she couldn't because she had to take Sasha to another medical appointment. And then I wanted a new (video game) for my birthday, and Mom said that we just couldn't afford it…I mean, I hear her on the phone talking about how she owes money and stuff to doctors and other people." The family therapist encouraged Patty to talk about how she felt, and helped Lorraine provide accurate and age appropriate, realistic information to Patty about Sasha's disorder, and the long-term time frame required for treatment. Once Patty was encouraged to discuss her feelings openly, she stopped instructing her sister to act out in school. The family therapist also helped Patti find a professional advocate and social worker at a community mental health agency. They helped her locate some private grants and funding for Sasha's treatment, as well as a free four week summer day camp program for children with autism in their neighboring county. Lorraine also was counseled to spend some special time alone with Patty.

The family therapist also encouraged Lorraine to join the local Autism Society of America chapter, and Patty was subsequently invited to a two week summer theater camp for neurotypical siblings of families with autism. Patty remarked in a later family session, "Yeah, after I met Marcy (another neurotypical girl with an autistic sibling) I liked her and then I heard her talking about how her brother would never lie, cheat, or steal…I guess I'm starting to figure out that Sasha might not play with me too well right now, but she's not so bad, I guess. Plus, she really is brave about all of her blood tests, and stuff. I don't think I would handle all of that as well as she does." This initial discovery of Sasha's positive features, brought about by expanding their immediate kin network, bode well for future family relationships and treatment.

Tommy was a 4 year-old boy diagnosed with autism. His parents recently moved, and were having difficulty finding a church that appeared accepting of their son's communication and behavioral issues. After seeking the assistance of a family therapist, Tommy's parents were encouraged to request a private meeting with their new pastor to discuss the situation proactively. After a series of successful meetings, the pastor encouraged Tommy's family to sit in the back of the church for regular Sunday services and quietly take their son in and out of the sanctuary if he became unable to sit still or quietly for the entire hour long service, rather than to miss the service or have to sit apart from one another.

With the parents' permission and direction, the pastor also took time during a church service to provide members of the congregation with general information about autism, and with specific information about how they could interpret some of Tommy's atypical behaviors (e.g., "If Tommy is flapping his hands and looking at the ground when you are talking to him, it doesn't mean he isn't listening. Right now, sometimes it helps Tommy if you speak softly or don't look directly at him when you speak to him…Tommy also may come up to you and put his arms around you; he does not yet understand that most of us have a kind of public space 'bubble' that we like to keep around ourselves. If he does put his arms around you, please know that he is doing that because even though he can't talk well yet, he likes you and wants to get to know you better. In that case, it is OK to gently take his arms from your shoulders and put them on your arm or gently on his own lap. We want to work together to help this family, so please ask Tommy's parents, Yvette and Armand, and me if there is anything you would like to know about Tommy or about autism.") The director of the church's youth group also worked closely with Tommy and his parents to find ways to successfully include him in activities and even a summer day camp.

Nicholas was a 3 year-old boy diagnosed with autism by his local intermediate unit after being "released" by three different day care centers for his aggressive and inappropriate behaviors (e.g., biting and pushing other children; screaming constantly; inability to attend during group activities; inability to play with toys appropriately). He also had significantly delayed and impaired speech, making it difficult to communicate. Both of Nicholas's parents worked full-time, and his father insisted that Nicolas "was just slow like most boys at talking and full of energy." Nicolas's mother, Priscilla, contacted a family therapist, after quitting her job and becoming depressed. The therapist met with Nicholas and his mother, Priscilla, for therapy sessions as Nicolas's father refused to attend. Nicholas had no aunts or uncles and his grandparents were deceased, so no immediate family was available for additional support.

The family therapist developed an action oriented treatment plan. She worked with Priscilla on dynamic issues related to her depression and her husband's denial. She also helped Priscilla connect with the local chapter of the Autism Society of America and similar organizations for help in acquiring ABA and other necessary therapies for Nicholas. The family's therapist also suggested that Priscilla seek out a foster grandparent. Priscilla was hesitant to pursue this plan at first, but after two weeks she asked an older woman in the neighborhood who had helped babysit Nicholas when he was younger. Priscilla was surprised and delighted when the older woman tearfully expressed her thanks to be involved, as her own young grandchildren lived far away and she had only limited contact with them.

Subsequently identified as "Nana," the older neighbor helped Priscilla with respite care, cooking, and companionship, and helped Nicholas with playing and his homework (i.e., ABA and speech therapy). Austra also helped coach Priscilla to be open and direct with "Nana" regarding both of their wishes for how much or how little time they wanted to spend together. For example, "Nana" indicated that she would be interested in babysitting Nicholas by herself once every other week, so that Priscilla could go on a much needed date night with her husband, but only when "Nana" felt comfortable enough with Nicolas to manage some of his tantrums. After a few months of treatment, one of Nicholas's first new words was "Nana," and along with some individual psychotherapy, Priscilla's depressive symptoms began to decrease. Taking the risk to expand the family system proved beneficial for everyone involved.

Conclusion

Family therapists can be called upon to expand their outreach and expertise to uniquely assist the approximately 1 in 46 families affected by a diagnosis of autism. Psychoeducation appears essential for both family members and clinicians (3,6), who can work as a unit to benefit not only the identified child but the entire family system. Just as family therapists can help affected parents and immediate family members expand their social network in creative ways for assistance, family therapists can be asked to help affected families and society as a whole by expanding their own professional role to include that of advocate. Only when family therapists, among other health care professionals, advocate for the rights of these underserved and typically overburdened families will appropriate national resources (e.g., guaranteed insurance benefits; funding for empirical research) be allocated for the treatment of childhood autism. With their understanding of dynamic systems and underlying psychological processes and disorders, family therapists are uniquely poised to assist these families in both crisis and the process of recovery.

Acknowledgment

This study was funded by the Pennsylvania State University, Berks research and development grant.

References

[1] Chakrabarti S, Fombonne E. Pervasive developmental disorders in preschool children. JAMA. 2001;24:3093-9.

[2] American Psychiatric Association. Diagnostic and statistical manual of mental disorders, 4th ed, text revision. Washington, DC: Author, 2000.

[3] Hillman J, Snyder J. Childhood Autism. New York: Routledge, 2007.

[4] U.S. Department of Health and Human Services. Mental health: A report of the Surgeon General. Rockville, MD: Author, 1999.
[5] Lovaas OI. Behavioral treatment and normal educational and intellectual functioning in young autistic children. J. Consult. Clin. Psychol. 1987;28:3-9.
[6] Hillman J. Supporting and treating families with children on the autistic spectrum: The unique role of the generalist psychologist. Psychotherapy. 2006;43:349-58.
[7] Gutstein S, Burgess A, Montfort K. Evaluation of the Relationship Development Intervention Program. Autism. 2007;11:397-412.
[8] Statistics Canada. Participation and activity limitation survey 2006: Families of children with disabilities in Canada. Ottawa, Canada: Social and Aboriginal Statistics Division, Statistics. Canada, 2006.
[9] Baker BL, McIntyre LL, Blacher J, Crnic K, Edelbrock C, Low C. Pre-school children with and without developmental delay: Behavioral problems and parenting stress over time. J. Intellect. Disabil. Res. 2003;47:217-30.
[10] Lecavalier L, Leone S, Wiltz J. The impact of behaviour problems on caregiver stress in young people with autism spectrum disorders. J. Intellect. Disabil. Res. 2006;50:172-83.
[11] Wiggs L, Stores G. Behavioural treatment for sleep problems in children with severe intellectual disabilities and daytime challenging behaviour: Effect on mothers and fathers. Br. J. Health Psychol. 2001;6:257-69.
[12] Davis NO, Carter AS. Parenting stress in mothers and fathers of toddlers with autism spectrum disorders: Associations with child characteristics. J. Autism Dev. Disord. 2008;38:1278-91.
[13] Koegel RL, Schreibman, L. Loos LM, Dirlich-Wilhelm H, Dunlap G, Robbins FR, et al. Consistent stress predictors in mothers of children with autism. J. Autism Dev. Disord. 1992;22:205–16.
[14] Rodrigue JR, Morgan SB, Geffken GR. Psychosocial adaption of fathers of children with autism, Down syndrome, and normal development. J. Autism Dev. Disord. 1992;22:249-63.
[15] Family Fund Trust. Statistical Analysis. York: Family Fund. 2003.
[16] Brennan EM, Brannan, AM. Participation in the paid labor force by caregivers of children with emotional and behavioral disorders. J. Emot. Behav. Disord. 2005;13:237-46.
[17] Kagan C, Lewis S, Heaton P. Combining work and care: Working parents of disabled children. York: Joseph Rowntree Foundation Findings, 1998.
[18] Orsmond G, Seltzer M. Siblings of individuals with autism or Down syndrome: Effects on adult lives. J. Intellect. Disabil. Res. 2007;51:682-96.
[19] Opperman S, Alant E. The coping responses of the adolescent siblings of children with severe disabilities. Disabil. Rehabil. 2003;25:441-54.
[20] Pit-Ten Cate I, Loots G. Experiences of siblings of children with physical disabilities: An emirical investigation. Disabil. Rehavil. 2000;22:399-408.
[21] Higgins DJ, Bailey SR, Pearce JC. Factors associates with functioning style and coping strategies of families with a child with an autism spectrum disorder. Autism. 2005;9:125-37.
[22] White N, Hastings RP. Social and professional support for parents of adolescents with severe intellectual disabilities. J. Appl. Res. Intellect. Disabil. 2004;17:181-90.
[23] Dunn ME, Burbine T, Bowers CA, Tantleff-Dunn S. Moderators of stress in parents ofchildren with autism. Community Ment. Health J. 2001;37:39-52.
[24] Knap JA. Raising a child with autism: The impact on the quality of marital relationships Dissertation. Minneapolis:MN: Walden Univ, 2005.
[25] Selgiman M, Goodwin G, Paschal K, Applegate A, Lehman L. Grandparents of children with disabilities: perceived levels of support. Educ. Train Ment. Retard. Dev. Disabil. 1997;32:293-303.
[26] Margetts JK, Le Courteur A, Croom S. Families in a state of flux: The experience of grandparents in autism spectrum disorder. Child Care Health Dev. 2006;32:565-74.
[27] Ferguson N, Douglas G, Lowe N. Grandparenting in divorced families. Bristol: Policy Press, 2004.
[28] Gray A. The changing availability of grandparents as carers and its implications for childcare policy in the UK. J. Soc. Policy. 2005;34:557-77.
[29] Hillman, J. Grandparents of children with autism: A review and recommendations for education practice, and policy. Educ. Gerontol. 2007;33:513-27.

[30] Findler LS. The role of grandparents in the social support system of mothers of children with a physical disability. Fam. Soc. 2000;81:370-81.

[31] Trute B. Grandparents of children with developmental disabilities: Intergenerational support and well-being. Fam. Soc. 2003;84:119-26.

[32] Baranowski M, Schilmoeller G. Grandparents in the lives of grandchildren with disabilities: Mothers' perceptions. Education and Treatment of Children. 1999;22:427-46.

[33] Wheelock J, Jones K. 'Grandparents are the next best thing': Informal childcare for working parents in Britain. J. Soc. Policy. 2002;31:441-63.

[34] Mirfin-Veitch B, Bray A, Watson M. 'They really do care': Grandparents as informal support sources for families of children with disabilities. N.Z. J. Disabil. 1996;2:136-48.

[35] Katz S, Kessel L. Grandparents of children with developmental disabilities: Perceptions, beliefs, and involvement in their care. Issues Compr. Pediatr. Nurs. 2002;25:113-28.

[36] Kolomer SR, McCallion P, Janicki MP. African-American grandmother carers of children with disabilities; Predictors of depressive symptoms. J. Gerontol. Soc. Work. 2002;47:45-63.

[37] Burnette D. Latino grandparents rearing children with special needs: Effects of depressive symptomatology. J. of Geron. Soc. Work 2000;33:1-16.

[38] Gardner JE, Scherman A, Efthimiadis MS, Shultz SK. Panamanian grandmothers' family relationships and adjustment to having a grandchild with a disability. Int. J. Aging Hum. Dev. 2004;59:305-20.

[39] Hayslip B, Kaminski PL. Grandparent raising their grandchildren: A review of the literature and suggestions for practice. Gerontologist. 2005;45:262-269.

[40] Burns C, Madian N. Experiences with a support group for grandparents of children with disabilities. Pediatr. Nurs. 1992;18:17-21.

In: Understanding Autism Spectrum Disorder
Editors: Ditza A Zachor and Joav Merrick

ISBN: 978-1-62081-353-9

Chapter 3

Best practices in the assessment and treatment of stereotypical behavior in individuals with autism

Kimberly N Sloman*[*], *Robert H LaRue*, *Mary Jane Weiss and Amy S Hansford

Douglass Developmental Disabilities Center, Rutgers, The State University of New Jersey, New Brunswick, New Jersey, US

Abstract

Stereotypy is one of the most prevalent problem behaviors for individuals with Autism Spectrum Disorders. Stereotypical behavior often occurs at high rates and interferes with the acquisition of skills, social interaction, and in some cases, may evolve into self-injurious behavior. The complex nature of stereotypical behavior can make the function difficult to assess and treatment development challenging. The purpose of this chapter is to review methods for interpreting the motivation (or function) of stereotypical behavior. Additionally, we provide an overview of behavioral treatment approaches for stereotypy maintained by automatic reinforcement.

Introduction

Individuals with autism engage in a variety of behaviors that are repetitive and non-functional. Often, these behaviors are described as stereotypical behaviors, or stereotypy. Stereotypical behaviors tend to occur at high rates and in many different contexts, and frequently appear to be unrelated to any other environmental events. These behaviors are described as part of the diagnostic features of autistic disorder (1).

---

[*] Correspondence: Kimberly N Sloman., PhD, Douglass Developmental Disabilities Center, Rutgers, The State University of New Jersey, 151 Ryders Lane, New Brunswick, NJ 08901 United States. Tel: (732) 932-3017 ; E-mail: ksloman@rci.rutgers.edu.

Stereotypy sets individuals with autism apart from their peers, and often makes social integration more challenging. At times, such behaviors may be stigmatizing from the perspective of peers, or may increase peer avoidance. In addition, these behaviors nearly always pose interference in learning. Individuals engaging in stereotypy are generally not attentive and may not be consistently responsive. For these reasons, stereotypic behaviors are often targeted for intervention. This chapter will review how stereotypy has been addressed, and will highlight the issues that exist regarding the assessment and treatment of these pervasive behaviors.

What is stereotypical behavior?

Stereotypy includes such behaviors as body-rocking, hand-gazing, hand-waving/flapping, finger flicking, noncontextual vocalizations, tongue clicking, and head-swaying and typically involves behavior that is rhythmic, repetitive, and high-rate. Topographical definitions of stereotypic behavior characterize it as repetitive motor and vocal responses (2,3).

While stereotypical behavior does occur during typical development (4,5), it tends to more prevalent in populations with developmental disabilities (6). Generally, stereotypical behavior that starts during childhood is more likely to persist if the individual has a developmental disability (7).

Such behaviors are primarily observed in people with developmental delay, especially those with a concurrent diagnosis of autism (8). Repetitive behavior, such as stereotypy, is a diagnostic indicator for autism (1,9). Since autism was first described in 1943, repetitive behavior has been a hallmark characteristic of the disorder (10). Several researchers have found that the incidence of stereotypical behavior is significantly higher in populations with autism than other developmental disabilities (11,12). In addition, researchers have found that the prevalence of stereotypy is directly correlated to the severity of autism symptoms. Although repetitive behavior is not specific to autism, the elevated pattern of occurrence and severity relative to other populations appears to characterize the disorder.

Why important to intervene?

While stereotypical behavior is often benign, certain topographies of behavior can become severe enough to produce tissue damage. Repetitive behavior, such as rocking, flapping arms, and finger posturing, can lead to internal injuries, scarring, or infection. In addition, several researchers have suggested that untreated stereotypical behavior can eventually lead to increased incidence of self injurious behavior (13,14).

Some studies have shown that when stereotypical behavior is interrupted, it can sometimes lead to an escalation in maladaptive behavior (15). Several studies have also shown that stereotypical behavior often interferes with skill acquisition (16-19). In addition, studies have also suggested that stereotypical behavior is stigmatizing and may interfere with social behavior (20). Furthermore, stereotypy is not likely to decrease without intervention (21-23). Jones (22) found that stereotypical behavior persisted for individuals at 10 year follow-ups for eight participants.

Factors affecting the occurrence of stereotypy

Stereotypical behavior is often defined by the fact that it often occurs in the absence of social consequences (24). In fact, stereotypical behavior is most often maintained by automatic reinforcement.

Several researchers have found that stereotypical behavior most commonly occurs during periods of low stimulation and "over-stimulation" (25). In other words, stereotypical behavior is most likely to occur in the absence of any stimuli to compete with the behavior or when stimulation is excessive (26,27). Lovaas, Newsom and Hickman (27) suggested that there are two primary causes of stereotypy. First, they suggested that stereotypy occurs in response to diminished environmental stimulation. In this scenario, the absence of stimulation is the motivating operation (MO) that establishes stimulation as a reinforcer, thus increasing the likelihood of the behavior (28,29). The second contributing factor is that stereotypical behavior may function as automatic negative reinforcement. Consequently, engaging in stereotypical behavior may reduce aversive stimulation (eg, an individual covering their ears and humming to diminish noise).

While most stereotypical behavior is maintained by automatic reinforcement, the behavior can come under the control of social reinforcement contingencies (30). Stereotypical behavior can be maintained by social positive reinforcement (access to sensory activities, tangible items or attention) and social negative reinforcement (escape from attention or demands). Given that stereotypical behavior tends to occur at high rates, the likelihood of adventitious reinforcement is high. In other words, the high frequency of the behavior increases the chance that social events, such as access to or escape from some stimulus, may inadvertently coincide with and begin to serve as reinforcement for the behavior. Thus, stereotypical behavior may be maintained specifically by the consequence the behavior itself produces or could be multiply maintained by both automatic and/or social reinforcement contingencies. This sensitivity of stereotypical behavior to social reinforcement contingencies has critical implications for treatment development and highlights the need for thorough functional assessments to accurately determine the function of the behavior.

Functional assessment of sterotypical behavior

As mentioned previously, the complexity of stereotypical behavior requires sound functional assessment procedures to accurately determine the function of the behavior and develop an effective intervention. The most empirically sound procedure for determining the operant mechanisms maintaining problem behavior is functional analysis (31).

Functional analyses generally involve the manipulation of specific antecedents and consequences for problem behavior. Conditions test for social positive reinforcement (eg, access to attention or tangibles), social negative reinforcement (eg, escape from demands or stimulation), and automatic reinforcement (i.e., behavior that persists in the absence of social consequences). These conditions are usually compared to an enriched environment (or control) condition. Each condition is presented for a set time period (eg, 10 minutes) and data are collected on rates or duration of problem behavior as well as potential motivating operations (eg, presence or absence of adult attention, demands, and preferred items).

Conditions are typically alternated in a multielement design and repeated until clear outcomes are observed.

In the social attention condition, attention is provided noncontingently and then withheld. Further attention is provided contingently upon the occurrence of problem behavior (eg, "Don't hit your head!"). If the individual engages in high rates of the behavior in this condition relative to control, social attention is implicated as a probable reinforcer.

In the tangible/restricted access condition, preferred items or activities are provided to the individual, withheld, and then represented contingent upon the target behavior. High rates of behavior in this condition relative to control indicate that problem behavior is maintained by access to tangible items.

The escape/demand condition is based upon the negative reinforcement paradigm; it determines if problem behavior is maintained by escape from an aversive stimulus. In this condition the individual is presented with a non-preferred stimulus (eg, difficult task), and the task is removed for 20-30 seconds contingent upon problem behavior. High rates of problem behavior in this condition relative to control suggest that escape from demands functions as reinforcement for the target behavior.

The alone/ignore condition is designed to evaluate the automatically reinforcing nature of the target behavior. This condition does not include programmed antecedents or consequences for target behavior. Traditionally, this condition is conducted with the individual placed in an empty room (i.e., alone). If there are concerns that the behavior is dangerous and may require an intervention, the condition may be conducted where the examiner is present but does not interact with the individual (i.e., ignore). If the individual engages in high rates of behavior in this condition it is likely that the behavior is reinforced by the natural consequences that the behavior itself produces (eg, sensory stimulation).

A toy play/control condition is the control to which all other conditions are compared. The individual is placed in an "enriched environment" in which he has access to preferred items, noncontingent attention, and an absence of demands/aversives. In this condition the examiner does not modify his behavior contingent upon the target behavior. If there is a clear external maintaining mechanism of problem behavior (i.e., attention, tangible, or escape) to problem behavior low rates are expected in this condition. High rates of problem behavior in the control condition lend support to an automatic function.

Patterns of automatically behavior

Hagopian et al. (32) outlined procedures for interpreting functional analyses. In their manuscript, Hagopian and colleagues documented several response patterns which are indicative of automatic reinforcement. The authors outlined three different patterns of automatically reinforced behavior in functional analyses.

The first pattern for automatically reinforced behavior is when the rate of behavior is high during the alone (or ignore) condition and relatively low during the other functional analysis conditions. This pattern suggests that the behavior is most likely to occur in the absence of others and is less likely to occur while others are present.

The second pattern for automatically reinforced behavior is when the rates of behavior are high in conditions with few items to compete (i.e., in conditions with less external stimulation), such as the alone, social attention, and tangible conditions and lower in the conditions with higher external stimulation (demand and control conditions).

The final pattern for automatically reinforced behavior is when the rates of behavior are relatively high and stable in all conditions. Frequent and relatively stable responding across conditions suggests that the source of reinforcement is present across time and conditions, which suggests that there is no functional relationship between the environmental manipulation and the behavior.

Extended alone manipulations

To clarify undifferentiated functional analyses (eg, similar rates of behavior in most or all conditions), extended alone conditions can help to confirm or rule out an automatic function for behavior (33). Vollmer and colleagues (33) suggested conducting multiple, consecutive alone sessions to help to rule out the possibility that behavior was maintained by social contingencies (eg, escape from the session room, inadvertent social reinforcement, multiple treatment interference). During extended alone conditions, sustained high rates of target behavior are suggestive of automatically reinforced behavior. If the rate of target behavior decreases over the course of sessions suggests that the behavior is socially mediated.

Analysis of within session responding

Changes in responding occur within sessions as a result of MO manipulations in the context of a functional analysis. Due to the presence or absence of an MO, the motivation to engage in certain behaviors changes (34,35). For instance, with behavior maintained by social positive reinforcement (eg, access to attention or tangibles), rates of maladaptive behavior are higher MO present (when access is restricted) than MO absent (while they have access to items/attention). For social negative reinforcement (eg, escape from aversive stimulation), rates of maladaptive behavior are higher MO present (while exposed to aversive stimuli) than MO absent (in the absence of aversive stimuli). When behavior is maintained by automatic reinforcement, the MOs manipulated are not necessarily relevant to the reinforcer maintaining the behavior. For automatically reinforced behavior, it is likely that the target behavior would occur at similar rates MO present and MO absent. In other words, another pattern would be high rates while the MO is present (eg, while social attention or preferred items were withheld, while instructions were provided) and high rates during periods when the MO is absent (eg, while they have access to attention or tangibles or during breaks).

In summary, functional analyses provide integral information on the maintaining consequences of behavior. More importantly, functional analyses are designed to directly prescribe treatments for inappropriate behavior. For example, if functional analysis results determine that problem behavior is maintained by escape from demands, a treatment can be developed in which (a) the aversiveness of the demand is lessened through reinforcer pairing, (b) the individual is taught an appropriate alternative response such as asking for a break, or (c) some combination of the two. The following section will provide an overview of behavioral treatments for stereotypy.

Behavioral treatment of stereotypic behavior

Although a small number of studies have demonstrated that stereotypy may be maintained by social reinforcement (30,36), the majority have shown that stereotypy persists in the absence of social consequences, or is automatically reinforced. The few studies which have identified that stereotypy is sensitive to social consequences serve as a reminder of the importance of functional analysis for a complete assessment and treatment approach. That is, it should not be assumed that behavior is automatically reinforced based on the topography alone. That being said, the focus of the treatment section will be on treatments for stereotypy that is maintained by automatic reinforcement.

Antecedent-based interventions

Environmental Enrichment/ Prompting. As previously discussed, a common functional analysis pattern of automatically reinforced behavior is high rates of the behavior only in conditions with little to no stimulation. In these cases, environmental enrichment may be an effective treatment. Environmental enrichment is a commonly used antecedent-based treatment for stereotypy. In practice, it allows free access to alternative sources of reinforcement in order to shift response allocation from stereotypy to the alternative items. These items are typically empirically selected via a variety of stimulus preference assessments (37). Briefly, these assessments determine preferences through direct observation of item engagement. That is, the items that the individual engages with the most are designated as the highest preferred. It should be noted that it is important to select items that are associated with high levels of engagement but low levels of stereotypy because previous research has shown that some high preference items may occasion high levels of stereotypy (18).

Numerous studies have demonstrated that simply providing competing sources of reinforcement in the form of preferred items to the individual is effective at reducing stereotypy (35,38-40). For example, Vollmer et al. (35) evaluated the effects on environmental enrichment with preferred and non-preferred items on the stereotypy of three individuals. Results showed that the presence of preferred items was necessary to reduce rates of stereotypy for all participants.

Other studies have shown that environmental enrichment is more effective when the included items match the putative sensory consequences of the specific topography of stereotypy (39, 41-44). For example, a radio may be indicated for vocal stereotypy while edible items may be indicated for hand mouthing. Piazza et al. (39) conducted duration-based stimulus preference assessments to determine high-preference items for each participant. The items were categorized as matched (i.e., items that produced similar sensory consequences to stereotypy) or unmatched (i.e., items that produced different sensory consequences to stereotypy). Results showed that the matched items produced greater decreases in stereotypy than unmatched items, even when the unmatched items were more preferred. In contrast, a recent study by Ahearn et al. (45) found that access to high preferred items, regardless of sensory properties, resulted in decreases in stereotypy. In addition, they argued that inclusion of a variety of reinforcers in environmental enrichment, not one sensory modality, would be beneficial to long-term treatment. The issue of matching the sensory consequences, therefore, is not entirely understood, and consensus has yet to be achieved. Nonetheless, it is widely accepted that access to preferred items can reduce stereotypy.

When access alone to alternative sources of reinforcement is not effective, other environmental adaptations may be necessary. A few studies have shown that providing periodic prompts to engage with the items is effective at reducing stereotypy (46). Others have shown that providing additional reinforcement for appropriate item interaction is necessary for effective treatment (35,47). For example, Favell et al. (47) demonstrated that environmental enrichment alone was ineffective at decreasing stereotypy. Specifically, the participants began to engage in stereotypy with the items. Stereotypy only decreased after additional reinforcement was provided for appropriate toy play.

In summary, environmental enrichment may be an effective and straightforward treatment of stereotypy for some individuals. This treatment may be particularly indicated when functional analysis patterns show low rates of the behavior in the control condition. However, previous research has shown that the methods used to determine alternative sources of reinforcement (eg, preferred and/ or matched sensory items) are integral in designing effective interventions.

Consequence-based interventions

Differential Reinforcement: Various forms of differential reinforcement have been used to treat stereotypy. During differential reinforcement a reinforcer may be provided for a) the absence of stereotypy for a set time interval (differential reinforcement of other behavior; DRO) b) an alternative response such as a request for an alternative sensory item (differential reinforcement of alternative behavior; DRA) or c) instances of stereotypy that occur after a period with no stereotypy (differential reinforcement of low-rate behavior; DRL). For example, Wacker et al (48) compared the effects of DRA to DRO in the treatment of stereotypic body rocking. In the DRA condition, the participant could request preferred and alternative sensory items. In the DRO condition, the same items were delivered for the absence of stereotypy for specified intervals. Both procedures were effective at decreasing stereotypy. Similarly, Taylor et al. (49) compared the effects of delivering preferred items using either DRO or a time-based, response-independent (noncontingent reinforcement, NCR) schedule of delivery on levels of stereotypy. Results showed that levels of stereotypy during the NCR condition were similar to baseline levels. In contrast, stereotypy decreased to low levels during the DRO condition. Additionally, stereotypy remained low as the schedule of reinforcement delivery was thinned. When some occurrences of stereotypy are permissible, a DRL schedule may be an appropriate treatment option. For example, Singh, Dawson, and Manning (50) provided social reinforcement for instances of stereotypy that occurred a set period of time from the last instance of stereotypy for three participants. Results showed that stereotypy decreased and appropriate social behavior increased. The efficacy of differential reinforcement procedures in the treatment of stereotypy has been replicated in numerous other studies (51,52).

Sensory Extinction/Response Blocking/Interruption: Sensory extinction involves the prevention or attenuation of the sensory consequences of stereotypy. Because stereotypy no longer produces those consequences, it diminishes over time. Sensory extinction is typically achieved by altering the environment (eg, padding the floors to attenuate the noise from stereotypic object banging) or providing protective equipment (eg, gloves for stereotypic hand rubbing). Several studies have investigated the effects of sensory extinction on stereotypy (53-56). For example, Rincover (56) evaluated the effects of various forms of sensory extinction on the stereotypy of three individuals. He found that extinction of specific sensory consequences was necessary to reduce levels of stereotypy. For example, in one case preventing the visual stimuli associated with stereotypy was not effective; however, preventing the auditory stimuli resulted in reduced rates of behavior. Therefore, when using sensory extinction it is important to assess which sensory aspects of the behavior are reinforcing to adequately implement the procedure.

Several studies have investigated the use of response blocking or response interruption on stereotypy. During these interventions, the individual is prohibited from engaging in stereotypy through physical blocking of the response (eg, guiding hands down for instances of hand flapping) or evoking an incompatible response (eg, providing a prompt to engage in vocal behavior for instances of vocal stereotypy). Response blocking/ interruption may result in decreases in stereotypy for two reasons. First, this procedure may capitalize on the sensory extinction of the stereotypy. That is, if the individual is prevented from engaging in the response and subsequently ceases to obtain sensory reinforcement, the response becomes less likely to occur. Second, the procedure may serve as punishment for engaging in stereotypy because the blocking/ interruption is aversive to the individual and therefore stereotypy decreases. Several studies have attempted to determine if response blocking serves as an extinction or punishment procedure (57-59). The results of these studies have indicated that the effects of response blocking may be idiosyncratic across individuals. That is, some studies have shown response patterns consistent with punishment effects (57) while others have shown response patterns consistent with sensory extinction (59).

Most studies utilizing response blocking/ interruption alone and in conjunction with other treatments are found to be highly effective at reducing rates of stereotypy (58,60-65). For example, Lindberg et al. (64) found that prompts to engage with competing items and prompts plus reinforcement for appropriate toy play were ineffective at reducing levels of stereotypy for two individuals. They evaluated response blocking and arm restraints and demonstrated decreases in stereotypy and increased rates of appropriate object manipulation. Similarly, Ahearn and colleagues (60) evaluated a response interruption and redirection (RIRD) procedure in the treatment vocal stereotypy for two participants. During RIRD, the therapist provided prompts to engage in an alternative vocal response contingent upon each occurrence of vocal stereotypy. Results showed that this procedure produced decreases in stereotypic vocalizations for both participants and increases in appropriate vocalizations for one participant.

Time Out/Response Cost: Recent studies have evaluated the use of negative punishment procedures such as time out or response cost in the treatment of stereotypy (61,66-67). These procedures are typically used when stereotypy persists in the presence of highly preferred items or activities. These items or activities are then removed for brief time intervals contingent upon stereotypy. For example, Falcomata et al. (66) found that access to preferred items alone was not effective at decreasing levels of stereotypy for one participant. However, stereotypy was reduced to low levels with the addition of a response cost component in the form of removal of a preferred item for 5-s continent upon stereotypy.

Conclusion

Stereotypy is a hallmark feature of individuals diagnosed with autism spectrum disorders. While stereotypy does not receive the same priority as behaviors that result in injury to self or others, they are socially significant. First, these behaviors often interfere with learning. They can impact attention, accuracy, speed, clarity and consistency of response. In addition, they can create social distance and stigmatization.

Assessment of stereotypy is imperative. While these behaviors often are automatically reinforcing, additional social functions are common. Functional analyses can yield useful information for treatment planning. Behavior analysts need to be familiar with the response patterns typically associated with an automatic reinforcement function. It is often useful to include additional assessment procedures, such as extended alone conditions, and analyzing within-session responding to clarify undifferentiated functional analyses to confirm or rule out an automatic function.

A variety of behavioral interventions have been shown to be effective in the treatment of automatically reinforced stereotypy. A common antecedent-based intervention is environmental enrichment, in which the individual is provided with alternative sources of reinforcement, which may serve as competition to the stereotypy. Although environmental enrichment has been demonstrated to decrease a wide-range of stereotypic behavior, research has shown that the efficacy is related to the type of stimuli selected for inclusion. Furthermore, several studies have shown that environmental enrichment may not be effective alone. Therefore, a comprehensive and effective treatment package may include additional treatments such as reinforcement of appropriate object manipulation, differential reinforcement procedures, sensory extinction, and response blocking to effectively reduce the behavior.

References

[1] American Psychiatric Association. Pervasive developmental disorders. In: Diagnostic and statistical manual of mental disorders, 4th ed, text rev (DSM-IV-TR). Washington, DC: Am Psychiatr Assoc, 2000:69-70.

[2] Matson JL, Kiely SL, Bamburg JW. The effect of stereotypies on adaptive skills as assessed with the DASH-II and Vineland Adaptive Behavior Scales. Res Dev Disabil 1997;18(6):471-6.

[3] Smith EA, Van Houten R. A comparison of the characteristics of self-stimulatory behaviors in "normal" children and children with developmental delays. Res Dev Disabil 1996;17(4):253-68.

[4] Foster LG. Nervous habits and stereotyped behavior in preschool children. J Am Acad Child Adolesc Psychiatr 1998;37(7):711-7.

[5] Tröster H. Prevalence and functions of stereotyped behaviors in nonhandicapped children in residential care. J Abnorm Child Psychol 1994;22(1):79-97.

[6] Berkson G, Rafaeli-Mor N, Tarnovsky S. Body-rocking and other habits of college students and persons with mental retardation. Am J Ment Retard 1999;104(2):107–16.

[7] Berkson G, McQuiston S, Jacobson JW, Eyman R, Borthwick S. The relation between age and stereotypic behaviors. Ment Retard 1985;23(1):31-3.

[8] Jones RSP, Walsh P, Sturmey P. Stereotyped movement disorders. London: Wiley, 1995.

[9] Lewis MH, Bodfish JW. Repetitive behavior in autism. Ment Retard Dev Disabil Res Rev 1998;4(2):80–89.

[10] Kanner L. Autistic disturbances of affective contact. Nervous Child 1973;2:217–50.

[11] Bodfish JW, Symons FJ, Parker, DE, Lewis, MH. Varieties of repetitive behavior in autism: Comparisons to mental retardation. J Autism Dev Disord 2000;30(3):237-43.
[12] Matson JL, Baglio CS, Smiroldo BB, Hamilton M, Packlowskyj T, Williams D, Kirkpatrick-Sanchez S. Characteristics of autism as assessed by the Diagnostic Assessment for the Severely Handicapped-II (DASH-II). Res Dev Disabil 1996;17(2): 135-43.
[13] Guess D, Carr E. Emergence and maintenance of stereotypy and self-injury. Am J Ment Retard 1991;96(3):299-319.
[14] Kennedy CH. Evolution of stereotypy into self-injury. In: Schroeder, SR, Oster-Granite, M, Thompson, T, eds. Self-Injurious Behavior: Gene-Brain-Behavior Relationships. Washington, DC, Am Psychol Assoc, 2002:133-43.
[15] Hagopian LP, Bruzek JL, Bowman LG, Jennett HK. Assessment and treatment of problem behavior occasioned by interruption of free-operant behavior. J Appl Behav Anal 2007;40(1):89-103.
[16] Dunlap G, Dyer K, Koegel RL. Autistic self-stimulation and intertrial interval duration. Am J Ment Defic 1983;88(2):194-202.
[17] Koegel RL, Covert A. The relationship of self-stimulation to learning in autistic children. J Appl Behav Anal 1973;5(4):381–7.
[18] Morrison K, Rosales-Ruiz J. The effect of object preferences on task performance and stereotypy in a child with autism. Res Dev Disabil 1997;18(2):127-37.
[19] Nijhof G, Joha D, Pekelharing H. Aspects of stereotypic behaviour among autistic persons: a study of the literature. Br J Dev Disabil 1998;44(1):3-13.
[20] Jones RSP, Wint D, Ellis NC. The social effects of stereotyped behaviour. J Intellect Disabil Res 1990;34(3):261-8.
[21] Horner RH, Carr EG, Strain PS, Todd AW, Reed HK. Problem behavior interventions for young children with autism: A research synthesis. J Autism Dev Disord 2002;32(50):423-46.
[22] Jones RSP. A 10 year follow-up of stereotypic behavior with eight participants. Behav Interventions 1999;14(1):45-54.
[23] Oliver C. Self-injurious behaviour in children with learning disabilities: Recent advances in assessment and intervention. J Child Psychol Psychiatr 1995;36(6):909-27.
[24] Vollmer TR. The concept of automatic reinforcement: Implications for behavioral research in developmental disabilities. Res Dev Disabil 1994;15(3):187-207.
[25] Repp AC, Karsh KG, Deitz DED, Singh NN. A study of the homeostatic level of stereotypy and other motor movements of persons with mental handicaps. J Intellect Disabil Res 1992;36(1):61-75.
[26] Hall S, Thorns T, Oliver C. Structural and environmental characteristics of stereotyped behaviors. Am J Ment Retard 2003; 108(6):391-402.
[27] Lovaas I, Newsom C, Hickman C. Self-stimulatory behavior and perceptual reinforcement. J Appl Behav Anal 1987;20(1):45–68.
[28] Michael J. Establishing operations. Behav Anal 1993;16(2):191-206.
[29] Laraway S, Snycerski S, Michael J, Poling A. Motivating operations and terms to describe them: Some further refinements. J Appl Behav Anal 2003;36(3):407-14.
[30] Kennedy CH, Meyer KA, Knowles T, Shukla S. Analyzing the multiple functions of stereotypical behavior for students with autism: implications for assessment and treatment. J Appl Behav Anal 2000; 33(4):559–71.
[31] Iwata BA, Dorsey MF, Slifer KJ, Bauman KE, Richman GS. Toward a functional analysis of self-injury. J Appl Behav Anal 1994;27(2): 197-209. (Reprinted from Anal Interv Dev Disabil 1982;2:3-20).
[32] Hagopian LP, Fisher WW, Thompson RH, Owen-DeSchryver J, Iwata BA, Wacker DP. Toward the development of structured criteria for interpretation of functional analysis data. J Appl Behav Anal 1997;30(2):313-26.
[33] Vollmer TR, Marcus BA, Ringdahl JE, Roane HS. Progressing from brief assessments to extended experimental analyses in the evaluation of aberrant behavior. J Appl Behav Anal 1995;28(4):561-76.
[34] Iwata BA, Pace GM, Kalsher MJ, Cowdery GE, Cataldo MF. Experimental analysis and extinction of self-injurious escape behavior. J Appl Behav Anal 1990;23:11-27.

[35] Vollmer TR, Marcus BA, LeBlanc L. Treatment of self-injury and hand mouthing following inconclusive functional analysis. J Appl Behav Anal 1994:27(2):331-44.

[36] Durand VM, Carr EG. Social influences on self-stimulatory behavior: Analysis and treatment application. J Appl Behav Anal 1987;20(2): 119-32.

[37] Cannella HI, O'Reilly MF, Lancioni GE. Choice and preference assessment research with people with severe to profound developmental disabilities: A review of the literature. Res Dev Disabil 2005;26(1):1–15.

[38] Mueller MM, Kafka C. Assessment and treatment of object mouthing in a public school classroom. Behav Interventions 2006;21(2): 137-54.

[39] Piazza CC, Adelinis JD, Hanley GP, Goh H, Delia MD. An evaluation of the effects of matched stimuli on behaviors maintained by automatic reinforcement. J Appl Behav Anal 2000;33(1):13-27.

[40] Ringdahl JE, Vollmer TR, Marcus BA, Roane HS. An analogue evaluation of environmental enrichment: The role of stimulus preference. J Appl Behav Anal 1997;30(2):203-16.

[41] Higbee TS, Chang S, Endicott K. Noncontingent access to preferred sensory stimuli as a treatment for automatically reinforced behavior. Behav Interventions 2005;20(3):177-84.

[42] Roberts-Gwinn MM, Luiten L, Derby KM, Johnson TA, Weber K. Identification of competing reinforcers for behavior maintained by automatic reinforcement. J Posit Behav Interv 2001;3(2):83-7.

[43] Sidener TM, Carr JE, Firth AM. Superimposition and withholding of edible consequences as treatment for automatically reinforced stereotypy. J Appl Behav Anal 2005;38(1):121-4.

[44] Tang J, Patterson TG, Kennedy CH. Identifying specific sensory modalities maintaining the stereotypy of students with multiple profound disabilities. Res Dev Disabil 2003;25:433-51.

[45] Ahearn WH, Clark KM, DeBar R, Florentino C. On the role of preference in response competition. J Appl Behav Anal 2005;38(2): 247-50.

[46] Britton LN, Carr JE, Landaburu HJ, Romick KS. The efficacy of noncontingent reinforcement as treatment for automatically reinforced stereotypy. Behav Interventions 2002;17(2):93–103.

[47] Favell JE, McGimsey JF, Shell RM. Treatment of self-injury by providing alternate sensory activities. Anal Interv Dev Disabil 1982; 2(1):83–104.

[48] Wacker DP, Steege MW, Northup J, Sasso G, Berg W, Reimers T, et al. A component analysis of functional communication training across three topographies of severe problem behavior. J Appl Behav Anal 1990;23(4):417–29.

[49] Taylor BA, Hoch H, Weissman M. The analysis and treatment of vocal stereotypy in a child with autism. Behav Interventions 2005; 20(4):239-53.

[50] Singh NN, Dawson MJ, Manning P. Effects of spaced responding DRL on the stereotyped behavior of profoundly retarded persons. J Appl Behav Anal 1981;14(4):521–6.

[51] Shabani D, Wilder D, Flood W. Reducing stereotypic behavior through self-monitoring and differential reinforcement of other behavior. Behav Interventions 2001;16(4):279-86.

[52] Miller BY, Jones RS. Reducing stereotyped behaviour: A comparison of two methods of programming differential reinforcement. Br J Clin Psychol 1997;36(3):297–302

[53] Rapp JT, Dozier CL, Carr JE, Patel MR, Enloe KA. Functional analysis of hair manipulation: A replication and extension. Behav Interventions 2000;15(2):121–33.

[54] Rapp JT, Miltenberger RG, Galensky TL, Ellingson SA, Long ES. A functional analysis of hair pulling. J Appl Behav Anal 1999;32(3), 329–37.

[55] Rapp JT, Miltenberger RG, Galensky TL, Ellingson SA, Long ES, Stricker J, Garlinghouse M. Treatment of hair pulling maintained by digital-tactile stimulation. Behav Ther 2000;31(2):381–93.

[56] Rincover A. Sensory extinction: A procedure for eliminating self-stimulatory behavior in developmentally disabled children. J Abnorm Child Psychol 1978;6(3):299–310.

[57] Lerman DC, Iwata BA. A methodology for distinguishing between extinction and punishment effects associated with response blocking. J Appl Behav Anal 1996;29(2):231–4.

[58] Mazaleski JL, Iwata BA, Rodgers TA, Vollmer TR, Zarcone JR. Protective equipment as treatment for stereotypic hand mouthing: Sensory extinction or punishment effects? J Appl Behav Anal 1994; 27(2):345-55.

[59] Smith RG, Russo L, Le DD. Distinguishing between extinction and punishment effects of response blocking: A replication. J Appl Behav Anal 1999;32(3):367–70.

[60] Ahearn WH, Clark KM, MacDonald RPF, Chung BI. Assessing and treating vocal stereotypy in children with autism. J Appl Behav Anal 2007;40(2):263-75.

[61] Athens ES, Vollmer TR, Sloman KN, Pipkin CSP. An analysis of vocal stereotypy and therapist fading. J Appl Behav Anal 2008;41(2): 291-7.

[62] Fisher WW, Lindauer SE, Alterson CJ, Thompson RH. Assessment and treatment of destructive behavior maintained by stereotypic object manipulation. J Appl Behav Anal 1998;31(4):513-27.

[63] Hagopian LP, Toole LM. Effects of response blocking and competing stimuli on stereotypic behavior. Behav Interventions 2009;24(2): 117-25.

[64] Lindberg JS, Iwata BA, Kahng S. On the relation between object manipulation and stereotypic self-injurious behavior. J Appl Behav Anal 1999;32(1):51-62.

[65] Symons F, Davis M. Instructional conditions and stereotyped behavior: The function of prompts. J Behav Ther Exp Psychiatr 1994; 25(4):317-24

[66] Falcomata TS, Roane HS, Hovanetz AN, Kettering TL, Keeney KM. An evaluation of response cost in the treatment of inappropriate vocalizations maintained by automatic reinforcement. J Appl Behav Anal 2004;37(1):83–7.

[67] Lerman DC, Iwata BA, Shore BA, DeLeon IG. Effects of intermittent punishment on self-injurious behavior: An evaluation of schedule thinning. J Appl Behav Anal 1997;30(2):187-201.

In: Understanding Autism Spectrum Disorder
Editors: Ditza A Zachor and Joav Merrick

ISBN: 978-1-62081-353-9

Chapter 4

Attachment among individuals with autism spectrum disorders

Nurit Yirmiya[1]*, Michal Shaked[1], Nina Koren-Karie[2] and David Oppenheim[3]

[1]Department of Psychology and School of Education,
The Hebrew University of Jerusalem, Mount Scopus, Jerusalem, Israel
[2]School of Social Work, University of Haifa, Mount Carmel, Haifa, Israel
[3]Department of Psychology, University of Haifa, Mount Carmel,
Haifa, Israel

Abstract

Attachment refers to the emotional tie that infants create with their caregivers. In the current review, we first introduce the reader to the concept of attachment and its measurement during childhood. Next, we offer an in-depth qualitative summary of the literature on attachment and autism. This growing body of studies reveals that children with autism spectrum disorders, just like children with other disabilities or with typical development, are able to form a secure attachment with the mother, although at a somewhat lower rate compared to typically developing children. We also present the associations among attachment and various characteristics of children along the autism spectrum (e.g., symptom severity, IQ) and mothers (i.e., sensitivity, resolution with diagnosis).

Introduction

Attachment refers to the emotional tie that infants create with their caregivers. The capacity and the desire to form close relationships are found in typically developing children from birth and are transformed into specific relationships with familiar caregivers by the end of the

* Correspondence: Nurit Yirmiya, PhD, Department of Psychology and School of Education, Hebrew University of Jerusalem, Mount Scopus, 91905 Jerusalem, Israel. E-mail: NYirmiya@gmail.com; NuritYirmiya@huji.ac.il

first year of life. Researchers have slowly begun to turn their attention to the study of attachment in children with various medical conditions and psychopathologies. Yet, the study of attachment and autism is in its infancy, most likely due to the once-held misconception that children with autism have no need or capacity to form attachments and/or that parents of children with autism actually contribute to the development of autism in their children through poor parenting. These notions, although no longer supported, may have held many professionals back from studying the experience of parenthood in parents of children with autism and their children's attachment. In the current review, we first introduce the reader to the concept of attachment and its measurement for typically developing children. Next, we offer an in-depth qualitative summary of the literature on attachment and autism. Finally, we present the associations among attachment and various characteristics of children along the autism spectrum (e.g., symptom severity, IQ) and mothers (i.e., sensitivity, resolution with diagnosis).

Attachment in typical development

John Bowlby (1-3) proposed that humans are biologically predisposed to form intimate relationships (attachments) and that development occurs within this interpersonal-relational matrix. Furthermore, these early relationships have long-lasting effects because they become part of the prototype for later relationships as well. Developmentally, Bowlby described four phases in the formation of attachment. The pre-attachment phase (age 0 to 6 weeks); the formation of attachment phase (6 weeks to 6-8 months); the attachment phase (6-8 months to 18-24 months); and the phase of creating internal models of relationships (from age 18-24 months and throughout life). Thus, in the first weeks and months of life, infants begin to respond selectively to people in contrast to objects, and begin to show a preference for their caregivers. However, only toward the age of 6 to 8 months do babies develop special relationships with their significant caregivers, and show greater comfort in the presence of the caregiver as well as a clear preference for the caregiver at times of stress.

Bowlby suggested that the attachment system is activated especially at times when infants are stressed, tired, or threatened; it is then that infants will show attachment behaviors such as actively seeking comfort from their attachment figures. Because infants have a basic need to become attached, forming an attachment to a significant caregiver is a universal phenomenon. Infants develop attachment relationships with any figure that provides consistent care regardless of the quality of that care, and will therefore develop attachments even toward an abusive or neglectful caregiver. Moreover, infants form attachments to more than just one caregiver, although at times of stress they will typically show a preference to their main attachment figure, if present (1,3). However, the quality of the attachment infants' form with each caregiver depends on the quality of the care they receive from the specific caregiver, and on the degree to which they have learned to view the attachment figure as a source of security and comfort.

On the basis of infants' daily experiences with the attachment figure during the first year of life, they develop a specific attachment pattern that Bowlby describes as either secure or insecure Securely attached infants feel free to explore thier surroundings, as they feels confident that the parent is available when needed. The reverse is the case with the insecurely attached infant, who cannot rely on his/her parent's physical and emotional availability and so lacks the emotional resources to effectively explore his environment.

Assessment of attachment patterns

Bowlby's theoretical perspective served as the basis for the development of a laboratory procedure called "The strange situation" (4,5). This procedure permits the observer to learn about the strategies that 12-18 month-old infants have developed for dealing with separation from their attachment figures and consequently about individual differences in the quality of attachment to their parents. This is achieved by examining the infant's behavior before, during and after a stressful situation involving exposure to a strange woman and two short separations from the parent (about three minutes each).

The procedure (4,6) consists of the following eight episodes: 1) Parent and infant are introduced to the experimental room (30+ seconds); 2) Parent and infant are alone. Parent does not participate while infant explores (three minutes); 3) Stranger enters, converses with parent, then approaches infant. Parent leaves inconspicuously (three minutes); 4) First separation episode: Stranger's behavior is geared to that of infant (three minutes or less if infant is distressed); 5) First reunion episode: Parent greets and comforts infant, then leaves again (variable); 6) Second separation episode: Infant is alone (three minutes or less); 7) Continuation of second separation episode: Stranger enters and gears behavior to that of infant (three minutes or less); 8. Second reunion episode: Parent enters, greets infant, sooth the child if needed; stranger leaves inconspicuously (variable).

The classification of children's attachment pattern is based mostly on the infant's behavior toward the parent during the reunion episodes. Behaviors such as proximity seeking, contact maintenance, resistance and avoidance permit the assessment of infants' ability to use their parent as a "secure base" from which they venture and explore the environment, and as a "haven of safety" to which they can return to gain comfort. Four types of infant attachment patterns can be identified using this procedure: Three traditional types of attachment, namely, Secure (B), Insecure- avoidant (A), and Insecure-ambivalent (C), and a forth type, Disorganized/ Disoriented (D) which was identified by Main and Solomon (7).

Securely attached infants (B) display a warm greeting of the parent following separation, and are able to utilize the parent as a source of solace and comfort. During the first part of the assessment, securely attached infants typically move away from their caregiver, yet they maintain eye contact while exploring their new surroundings. When the mother returns, if the infants were distressed, they typically seek immediate contact, which is effective in relieving and terminating the distress. If they were not distressed, they show clear signs of happiness upon the mother's return by actively greeting her and initiating interaction with her. Insecure-Avoidant attached infants (A-Type) usually exhibit no overt symptoms of stress or discomfort when the parent leaves the room. They readily separate from her and are affiliative toward the stranger both in mother's presence and in her absence. Upon the mother's return, they may avoid her and show no awareness of her return and make no attempt to seek contact or interaction with her. One may assume that these children are securely attached because they do not demonstrate overt stress. However, physiological measures of stress (such as heart rate and levels of cortisol in the blood) clearly show that these children are extremely stressed in the Strange Situation (8), but have learned to repress the external behavioral manifestation of that inner stress.

Winnicott (9) referred to this state of self as a false self, because the child adapts a compliant behavioral state that s/he perceives as desired by the caregiver, but the child does not express the true self, which in this case would be revealing the inner stress. The Insecure-Ambivalent attached (C-type) infants are characterized by extreme stress during separation from the parent. At the same time, they are unable to calm down and return to exploratory activity upon reunion, and their proximity-seeking behavior is combined with resistant behavior.

In normative samples consisting of typically developing children between the ages of 1 and 2 years, about 65% of the children revealed secure attachments (B), 20% received a classification indicating an insecure-avoidant attachment style (A), and about 15% were classified with an insecure-anxious attachment style (C) (10). The A, B, and C patterns of attachment reflect coherent (although not necessarily adaptive) strategies adopted by infants towards their attachment figures upon activation of the attachment system. While A and C attachment patterns may represent risk factor in infants development, it must be emphasized that these classifications are in no way signs of psychopathology.

The fourth category of attachment, Insecure-disorganized (identified by the letter D), characterizes children who do not show a consistent pattern of behavior in the strange situation, or show momentary breakdowns in their coping strategy, manifested by a confused and even contradictory array of responses (7). This category was added later based on observations of about 200 infants from various laboratories who could not be classified into any of the three aforementioned classifications, because they did not manifest an organized strategy of dealing with stress in the presence of their caregiver (7, 11).

These children may at times display contradictory attachment behaviors, expressions of fear toward the parent, stereotypies, undirected movements, and freezing.

These disorganized behaviors appear as momentary breakdowns in a dominant strategy, and thus the category D is assigned along with an additional coding given to identify the secondary pattern (A, B, or C). Altogether, about 15% of typically developing children receive this additional classification of D (12).

Mother as secure base

Home observations (13) targeting dyads of mothers and their infants in the last quarter of the first year of life indicated differences in maternal behaviors between mothers of infants classified as A vs. B vs. C. Mothers of infants classified as securely attached (B) were the most sensitive in responding to their infant's signals and communications. These mothers could see things from the baby's point of view, and they responded contingently, promptly, and appropriately. When these mothers did not give their infants what they seemed to desire, the mothers did so tactfully by acknowledging and offering an alternative. These mothers were accessible, accepting, and non-interfering.

Mothers of insecurely attached infants revealed less sensitive parenting compared to mothers of securely attached infants. However, maternal insensitivity did not differentiate between the two classifications of mothers of insecure infants, those with insecure-anxious

(C) versus insecure-avoidant (A) attachment patterns. What differentiated these two groups was the mother's degree of rejection: Mothers of children with an insecure A pattern displayed more rejecting behaviors than mothers of children with an insecure C pattern. Mothers whose infants received the C classification were not conspicuously rejecting of their infants. Most of them were found to play with their children, and were affectionate toward the infant occasionally. However, they were insensitive, by either mostly ignoring their child or by interfering (14).

Home observations demonstrated that, compared to infants with an insecure attachment pattern (A or C), infants with a secure attachment (B) were less anxious in everyday separations, more often initiated being picked up, were soothed more easily by body contact, responded more positively to being picked up and held, sought less to be put down, cried less overall, tended to greet their mothers positively upon the mothers' return, and were more willing to be put down after being held. In contrast to the securely attached (B) infants, the infants with an insecure attachment pattern (A or C) showed more distress at home by crying more overall, crying more when mothers returned after typically short separations throughout the day, and responding less positively to physical contact. The comparison between the two insecure attachment patterns at home indicated that infants with an avoidant classification (A) were angrier and were less accepting of mothers' physical holding than infants with an anxious (C) attachment pattern.

Observations of the mothers of infants with A versus C attachment patterns also revealed clear differences (13, 15). Mothers of infants with an avoidant (A) attachment pattern tended to reject physical contact and were angrier and more compulsive than mothers of infants with an anxious (C) classification.

Mothers of infants with an anxious attachment were not rejecting, and they actually seemed to enjoy physical contact, but they were still less sensitive compared to mothers of infants with a secure attachment. Thus, it appeared that because mothers of infants with an anxious attachment pattern were insensitive, these babies, in turn, experienced conflict regarding their mothers' responsiveness due to their learned expectation that they would be frustrated. A different story emerged for infants with an avoidant attachment pattern. These infants seemed to have learned that their mothers rebuffed them, and, thus, although wanting closeness and contact, they learned to avoid it so that they would not experience rejection (13, 15).

The benefits of having a secure attachment have been shown over and over with typically developing children. Reports revealed that children who were securely attached in infancy exhibited better mentalizing abilities concurrently as well as at later ages (i.e., symbolic play, theory of mind, and understanding of emotions) compared to children who received insecure classifications in infancy (16-18). Also, security of attachment was found to be associated with the children's more advanced linguistic abilities, more advanced mental states (19,20), and better general social and emotional adjustment (21-23).

Autism provides an interesting field in the context of attachment theory because of the significant and pervasive impairments in the social and communication skills of children with autism, as well as in their capacity to initiate interaction and engagement with others. Yet, as attachment theory predicts that maternal behavior is the antecedent of attachment security, it is important to investigate whether children with autism respond selectively to their mothers and form secure attachments with them in a similar way to typically developing children. In the next section, we will describe the studies available pertaining to attachment and autism.

Attachment and autism

Working at UCLA, Marian Sigman and her research group have been involved in studying the attachment of young children with autism. Sigman and Ungerer's (24) examination of 14 children with autism revealed these children's dramatic increase in mother-directed proximity-seeking during reunion compared to their behavior prior to separation. The fact that no such behavior was found toward the stranger in the room indicates these children's clear attachment responses to their mothers. To tease out possible influences of age and IQ, Sigman and Mundy (25) compared the behaviors of the same group of 14 children with autism (mean age of four years, three months; mean mental age of two years) to the behaviors of two other groups: a clinical group matched on chronological and mental age, and a much younger group of typically developing children matched only on mental age. The clinical group consisted of children with developmental delay having a mean age of five years and a mean mental age of 2 years, 2 months. The typically developing children had a mean age of 1 year, 8 months and a mean mental age of 2 years. During separation from the caregiver in the strange situation, the typically developing group showed more distress leading to episode termination, thus resulting in a significantly shorter separation episode for this group compared to the two clinical groups. However, other than duration, no other significant differences were found for any of the behaviors (corrected to reflect percentage of time scores) during the separation episode. During the reunion episode, no significant behavioral differences emerged between the children with autism and the children with a developmental delay, although both clinical groups differed from the typically developing children who were more involved with their caregiver. Yet, importantly, all 14 children with autism, 11 of the 14 children with developmental delay, and 12 of the 14 typically developing children interacted much more with the caregiver than with the stranger during the reunion episode.

Sigman and Mundy (25) conducted a replication study with a larger sample of three groups: children with autism (chronological age of 4 years, 5 months; mental age of 2 years, 2 months), children with developmental delay (chronological age of 4 years, 2 months; mental age of 2 years, 2 months), and children with typical development (chronological age of 1 year, 10 months; mental age of 2 years, 1 months). For this sample, the separation episodes had to be terminated for 5 typically developing children and for 3 children with autism during the first separation episode, and for 7 typically developing children, 4 children with autism, and 1 child with developmental delay during the second separation episode. Furthermore, the typically developing children as a group were more distressed during the first separation than either clinical group, who did not differ from each other. During the second separation, the typically developing children were again more distressed than either clinical group, but this time the group with autism was also significantly more distressed than the group of children with developmental delay.

During both reunions, all three groups of children directed more social behavior toward the mother than toward the stranger, and the typically developing children directed significantly more social behavior toward their mothers compared to each of the two clinical groups. In the first reunion, the two clinical groups did not differ from each other in their social behavior toward the mother; however, it is important to note that during the second reunion, the children with autism displayed significantly more social behavior toward the mother compared to the children with developmental delays.

In the next study from UCLA, Capps, Sigman, and Mundy (26) actually classified the attachment patterns of children with autism using the Ainsworth system. They found that although all of the children (chronological age: 4 years; mental age: 2 years) displayed disorganized behavior that was probably associated with their autism, 6 of the 15 children (40%) received a secondary classification of secure attachment (B). Of the remaining 9 children who received a secondary classification of insecurity, only 3 received a "true" D classification, suggesting disorganized, confused behaviors other than those associated with autism. Two children received a classification of insecure-ambivalent (C), 1 child received a classification of insecure-avoidant (A), and the remaining 3 could not be classified because they manifested confusing signs of security and insecurity. The UCLA group concluded that, altogether, children with autism form secure attachments to their mothers at rates resembling those of other children.

Shapiro et al (27) examined the attachment organization of 15 children with autism (chronological age: 3 years, 4 months; mean DQ = 64.8) compared to 10 children with pervasive developmental disorder (PDD; mean chronological age: 3 years, 8 months; mean DQ = 80), 8 children with developmental language disorders (mean chronological age: 3 years, 4 months; mean DQ = 79), and 3 children with developmental delay (mean chronological age: 4 year, 2 months; mean DQ = 41). These researchers found that 8 of the 15 children with autism, 5 of the 10 children with PDD, 1 of the 8 children with a language disorder, and 1 of the 3 children with developmental delay were classified as securely attached, once more emphasizing that the rate of secure attachments in children with autism is comparable to that in the general population.

Rogers, Ozonoff, and Maslin-Cole (28) compared the attachment security of 17 children with autism or PDD (mean chronological age of 4 years 3 months; mean IQ of 85) with that of 17 children with psychiatric difficulties other than autism (reactive attachment disorder, oppositional disorder, adjustment disorder, developmental delay; mean chronological age of 4 years; mean IQ of 83). Using a modification of the strange situation and its coding, these researchers reported that a comparable distribution of secure and insecure assignments was found in the two groups. In their next publication, Rogers et al (29) reported on a larger and slightly younger sample of 32 children with autism or PDD (mean chronological age of 3 years, 10 months; mean IQ of 72). Of these 32 children, 12 (37.5%) showed secure attachments, and 4 others (12.5%) showed signs of security that were as strong as their nonsecurity signs. Thus, the authors concluded that 50% of the children with autism in their sample revealed signs of security that were at least equivalent to, or predominated over, signs of insecurity.

Dissanayake and Crossley (30,31) examined the behavior of 16 children with autism (mean chronological age: 4 years, 4 months), 16 children with Down syndrome (mean chronological age: 4 years, 7 months), and 16 typically developing children (mean chronological age: 4 years 3 months) during several episodes similar to those employed in the strange situation. First, mother and child were together in the room, then a stranger entered, and the child remained with both adults. Next, the mother left, and then she returned. Analyses of discrete behaviors revealed that although children with autism were less social toward their mothers compared to the two other groups, in the first episode when they were with her in the playroom, once the experimenter entered the room, all children sought and maintained proximity to their mothers. Similarly, overall, the behavior of children with autism during the separation and reunion episodes was similar to that of the other two groups.

The lack of significant differences between the groups suggests that children with autism, just like other children, use their mothers as a secure base.

Spencer (32) investigated the attachment behaviors of 20 children with autism (mean chronological age of 2 years, 6 months; mean mental age of 1 year, 4 months), 20 children with developmental delays (a mixed group of children with Down syndrome, Fragile X syndrome, cerebral palsy, and unknown etiology; mean chronological age of 2 years, 3 months; mean mental age of1 year, 4 months), and 20 young children with typical development (mean chronological age of 1 year, 3 months; mean mental age of 1 year, 4 months). Compared to other studies, Spencer's study focused on younger children. Examination of the children's behaviors during one separation and one reunion episode revealed more similarities than differences among the groups. First, no significant group differences emerged in length of the separation episode, which contrasted to Sigman et al (25), who found shorter episode length for the typically developing children given their strong reaction to the separation. Second, no significant differences emerged among the groups with regard to the distribution of children within each group who were not upset, who comforted themselves, or who allowed the examiner to soothe them. Third, no significant group differences appeared in the number of children who immediately oriented to the mother's leaving or who appeared not to notice that the mother left. Differences emerged only in behaviors relating to the overall focus of the child during separation: Most of the children with developmental delays or typical development responded by interacting with the examiner, whereas half of the group of children with autism preferred to maintain solitary behaviors. Furthermore, 5 of the children with autism actively searched for their mother, a behavior that was not revealed by any of the children in the other two groups.

For several behaviors during reunion (32), significant differences emerged only between the group of children with autism and the group with typical development. First, 13 of the 20 children with autism compared to 15 of the 20 children with developmental delay and 18 of the 20 typically developing children approached their mother and requested contact or touched them. Second, only 5 of the children with autism, 4 of the children with developmental delay, and 1 of the typically developing children did not respond immediately to their mother upon her return. Third, only 3 children with autism, in contrast to 8 children with developmental delay and 14 children with typical development, actively attempted to maintain proximity with the mother upon her return. Thus, children with autism did not differ in these attachment behaviors during reunion from other children with developmental delays. Furthermore, no significant group differences emerged for patterns of behaviors relating to soothability and resistance during reunion but did emerge for an overall global qualitative summary score. Spencer concluded that children with autism do form attachments, although their behaviors differ somewhat from those of other children. This study's findings of similarities and differences in the discrete attachment behaviors of children with autism once more indicate the difficulty inherent in teasing out behaviors indicating attachment from the social and communicative behaviors inherent in autism.

In the Netherlands, Willemsen-Swinkels et al (33) examined 32 young children with autism or PDD, with moderate to severe autism (mean chronological age of 68.2 months; mean mental age of 42.2 months), 19 children with expressive or receptive language disorders (mean chronological age of 63 months; mean mental age of 53 months), and 19 children with typical development (mean chronological age of 54 months; mean mental age assumed to equal chronological age). The group with autism was further divided into 13 low-functioning children (mean chronological age of 67 months; mean mental age of 2 years) and 19 high-functioning children (mean chronological age of 69 months; mean mental age of 55 months). Findings demonstrated the highest D classification in the low-functioning group with autism (53.8%; 7 of the 13), whereas a D classification was given only to 16.7% (3 of the 19) of the high-functioning children with autism, only to 15.8% (3 of the 19) children with language disorders, and 10.5% (2 of the 19) of the children with typical development. When examining the distribution of the A, B, and C classifications, no significant differences emerged among the groups in the proportion of securely attached children (B): 78.9% for typical development, 84.2% for language disorders, 66.7% for high-functioning PDD, and 54% for low-functioning PDD. Similarly, the percentages of securely attached children in the autism and PDD not otherwise specified (PDD-NOS) groups were similar (63.6% and 62.5%, respectively). It is important to note that, similarly to typically developing children who received a classification of D (34), children diagnosed with PDD who were classified D also revealed an elevated heart rate during separation and reunion with their mothers, thus indicating their greater stress compared to peers who were not classified as D.

In 2004, the Netherlands group collected all the published studies on attachment and autism and conducted a meta-analytic study (35). These researchers asked the following questions: Do children with autism have the same chance as children without autism to form a secure attachment relationship with their parents? What are the associations between security of attachment on the one hand and mental development and chronological age on the other hand in children with autism? Furthermore, these researchers were interested in exploring possible differences in attachment security between children diagnosed with PDD-NOS and those diagnosed with autistic disorder, and whether the experimental designs in which the groups were matched differed from those in which the groups were not matched.

The meta-analysis revealed that children with autism do form secure attachments with their mothers, but that compared to children without autism (i.e., one group containing both typically developing children and children with mental retardation and other psychopathologies), children with autism scored about one-half of a standard deviation lower on attachment security. Furthermore, studies in which the participants were diagnosed with autistic disorder yielded larger effect sizes compared to studies in which the participants were diagnosed with PDD-NOS. That is, larger differences in attachment security emerged from the comparison of children diagnosed with autism to other children than from the comparison of children diagnosed with PDD-NOS to other children. Similarly, larger differences in attachment security emerged from the comparison of low-functioning children with autism to other children than from the comparison of high-functioning children with autism to other children. Significant differences emerged only between the low-functioning group with autism and the comparison groups. Finally, chronological age, matching (matched versus unmatched designs), and year of publication were not found to be associated with findings regarding attachment security in this meta-analysis (35).

In sum, when all children with autism from all studies were pooled together (35) the meta-analysis data showed that children with autism were able to form secure attachments. However, their finding of a security index 0.5 SD below that of the comparison group should be considered cautiously in view of the heterogeneous single comparison group used. By pooling together children with a language disorder or with mental retardation as well as other etiologies, along with normative samples of 12- to 21-month-old infants, with no further differentiation based on etiology, age, symptoms, etc., the meta-analysis results are somewhat inconclusive as it remains unclear as to whether children with autism actually receive lower security scores compared to each of these subgroups. Furthermore, the authors made a decision that whenever a report on children with autism did not involve a comparison group (for example,(26)), they compared the results to large normative samples of typically developing infants who did not actually participate in autism research.

A recent longitudinal research program by the Netherlands group further explored attachment behaviors in children with autism as compared to children with or without developmental difficulties. These studies involve a population-based sample recruited from around 30,000 children participating in a screening study in the province of Utrecht (36,37). The advantage of a longitudinal study is that the children were recruited at a young age, enabling the use of the classic strange situation paradigm described above, as opposed to modified versions employed in other studies with older children. The first publication from this study (38) reported on the attachment classifications of five groups of children at age 14 months: 20 toddlers with autistic disorder, 14 toddlers with PDD, 12 toddlers with mental retardation, 16 toddlers with language disorders, and 18 typically developing toddlers. Results revealed a significant difference in attachment classification distribution between the non-clinical and clinical groups: Children with a developmental disorder were less often securely attached than the typically developing children. No significant differences in distribution of secure versus insecure assignments emerged between the four clinical groups. Regarding the assignment of disorganized attachment patterns, the attachment pattern of the children in all clinical groups was more often disorganized than in the typical group. Furthermore, a disorganized attachment style was associated with a relatively lower developmental level (mental abilities) even more than it was associated with the severity of autistic symptoms.

In an ensuing publication from this research program (39), the researchers employed the Brief Attachment Q-Sort (40) based on the Attachment Q-Sort (41) to conduct naturalistic observations of parent-child interactions, emphasizing secure-base behavior. It consists of cards with specific behavioral descriptions, and can be used with children as old as 48 months. The BASQ contains 12 items with high loadings on the security scale. This study (39) compared 25 high-functioning children with autism spectrum disorder (ASD), 16 low-functioning children with ASD, 12 children with mental retardation, 11 children with language disorders and 25 typically developing children. Results showed that the combined group of high- and low-functioning children with ASD showed significantly less attachment security than the non-clinical comparison group.

In other recent research, Oppenheim and colleagues (42) working in Israel examined the attachment security of 45 young boys with autism (mean age of 4 years, 1 month) using the strange situation procedure. Findings indicated that 19 children were classified as securely attached, 16 children were classified as anxiously attached (7 ambivalent and 9 avoidant), and 10 children were classified with disorganized attachment.

In contrast to the aforementioned studies that involved relatively young children with autism, Taylor, Target, and Charman (43) were the first and so far the only researchers who examined attachment in high-functioning adults with autism (n = 5) and Asperger Syndrome (n = 15) between the ages of 19 and 60 years (M = 34 years). Employing the Adult Attachment Interview (44), these researchers found that only 3 of the 20 participants (15%) revealed a secure model of attachment, indicating a lower rate compared to non-clinical samples but one similar to other clinical adult samples. The remaining 17 participants received a classification of either "preoccupied," (characterized by being preoccupied with or by past attachment relationships or experiences (n=8), or "dismissing," which is characterized by talking about past attachment relationships as lacking an influence on later life, emotions and adult personality (n=9).

One final study has relevance to our understanding of attachment security in children with autism, although it differed somewhat in that attachment was assessed by maternal perceptions only. Hoppes and Harris (45) studied the perceptions of 17 mothers of children with autism (chronological age: 7 years) and 21 mothers of children with Down syndrome (chronological age: 9 years). Using a questionnaire to ask mothers about their perceptions of their children's attachment, the researchers found that mothers of children with autism reported significantly less perceived attachment as well as significantly less maternal gratification compared to the mothers of children with Down syndrome. This is the only study that actually asked mothers about their perceptions of their children's attachment security. However, the study lacked a comparison group of typically developing children and their mothers; therefore, the findings of greater perceived attachment in the Down syndrome group may possibly stem from the well-known very high sociability of these children and may not necessarily predict such differences between mothers of children with autism and with typical development. Indeed, most of the aforementioned studies indicate that the attachment of children with autism to their caregivers is more similar to than different from that of other children, suggesting that the mothers of children with autism may not differ in their perceptions from mothers of typically developing children. Finally, although this study did not include direct assessments of attachment, it suggests that mothers of children with autism may experience more difficulties in perceiving, understanding, and interpreting the attachment behaviors of their children.

Correlates of attachment security and insecurity

As can be seen from the review so far, clearly children with autism form attachments with their caregivers, with about 50% of them forming secure attachments with the caregivers. Various researchers have examined whether different child and maternal variables are associated with attachment security and insecurity in autism. In this section, we review correlates such as the child's symptom severity, verbal ability, age, or IQ and maternal representations and behaviors.

Play behavior

In their first study, Sigman and Ungerer (24) found that the duration and diversity of symbolic play was significantly associated with positive reunion behaviors as defined in their study. Children with autism who interacted more with their mothers during reunion showed longer and more diverse symbolic play. Play diversity clearly distinguished children with autism who did or did not show a clear response to their mothers' departure and return. However, in their second study with the same children, this finding was not replicated (25).

Likewise, Naber et al (38) reported an association between children's quality of play behavior and their attachment. In particular, those children from all groups who were classified as secure using the strange situation procedure showed higher levels of play compared to children classified as insecure. In contrast, Marcu et al (46) found that children with secure attachment did not score higher on measures of symbolic play compared to children with insecure attachments (insecure-avoidant, insecure-ambivalent, and insecure-disorganized). However, children with organized attachments (secure, insecure-avoidant, and insecure-ambivalent) did score higher on measures of symbolic play compared to children with disorganized attachment. These inconsistent findings may be associated with different approaches to coding symbolic play as well as various methodologies of grouping participants.

Mental age

Sigman and Ungerer (24) and Sigman and Mundy (25) found no association between attachment security and mental age. Likewise, Capps et al (26) did not find an association between attachment classification and intelligence. Similarly, Shapiro et al (27) found no differences on DQ between children with autism who were classified as securely attached and those classified as insecurely attached. Finally, Taylor et al (43) did not find an association between attachment classification based on the Adult Attachment Interview and IQ in their sample of high functioning adults.

On the other hand, some studies indicated a possible association between attachment and mental age. Rogers et al (28,29) found an association between their attachment security measure and cognitive abilities (not IQ). Willemsen-Swinkels et al (33) reported a lower rate of secure attachment among low-functioning children with autism and PDD-NOS in comparison to their high-functioning counterparts. In the study by Naber et al. (38), children with mental retardation were less often classified as securely attached than children without mental retardation. Oppenheim et al (42) also found that attachment and IQ were associated in that insecure/disorganized children were more likely to be low-functioning, whereas insecure/organized and secure children were more likely to be high-functioning. Inconsistent findings may be due to the fact that some researchers coded attachment into 4 categories (secure insecure ambivalent, insecure avoidant and disorganized) whereas others used the first three categories only, and did not code disorganized attachment.

Chronological age

Whereas Sigman and Ungerer (24), Sigman and Mundy (25), and Oppenheim et al (42) did not find an association between attachment and chronological age, Hoppes and Harris (45) as well as Rogers et al (29) found an association between attachment security and chronological age, in that higher attachment security was associated with children's older ages. It is important to note that these differences may be associated with different methodologies in that the Rogers study did not use the attachment classifications system and Hoppes assessed only maternal perceptions.

Language

Sigman and Mundy (25) did not find an association between children's attachment security and their language abilities. However, most other research showed significant associations in this regard. For example, Capps et al (26) reported that the language abilities of children with a secure attachment were significantly higher than the language abilities of children who were insecurely attached.

Likewise, Dissanayake and Crossley (31) found that children with autism who were verbal reacted with more intensity in the reunion episodes compared to children with autism who were nonverbal. Rogers et al (28) also found an association between their attachment security measure and language abilities in that higher attachment security was associated with better language abilities among children.

Finally, the one study of high-functioning adults with autism and Asperger disorder (43) pinpointed a negative correlation between the communication scale score on the well-known Autism Diagnostic Observation Schedule (ADOS) and the narrative coherence scale of the Adult Attachment Interview.

Nonverbal communication

Capps et al (26) reported that children who were securely attached displayed significantly more looking, pointing, and giving to obtain help from their mothers, and were more responsive to the experimenter, compared to children with an insecure attachment classification. Similarly, Willemsen-Swinkels et al (33) and Koren-Karie et al (47) found that securely attached children with autism and PDD initiated more socially, were more responsive to the parent and involved them more compared to insecurely attached children.

Autism symptom onset and severity

Rogers et al (29) and Oppenheim et al (42) found no association between attachment and severity of autism. Nor did group differences emerge between PDD and autism regarding attachment security in that study, even though the PDD group had higher social and language scores and fewer symptoms. Similarly, Willemsen-Swinkels et al (33) did not find differences between children diagnosed with autism and children diagnosed with PDD-NOS. Likewise, Shapiro et al (27) found no differences between children with autism who were classified as securely attached and those classified as insecurely attached, nor between children diagnosed with autism and children diagnosed with PDD.

Conversely, Rogers and Dilalla (48) found that the attachment security of children with an onset of autistic symptoms between 12 to 24 months was significantly lower than that of children with symptom onset after age 24 months. They also reported lower attachment security scores for children diagnosed with autism compared to children diagnosed with PDD. Naber et al (38) also found a correlation between severity of autism symptoms as assessed in the ADOS and insecure attachment assignments. In another publication from this research project (49), less severe autistic symptoms in the social domain predicted more attachment security.

Maternal representations and sensitivity

As in samples of typically developing children (50), Capps et al (26) found that mothers of securely attached children with autism tended to be more sensitive when interacting with their children than mothers of insecurely attached children. Pechous (51) investigated attachment in young children with autism who were receiving 25 to 40 hours per week of an intensive behavioral intervention focused on communication and social/emotional abilities. The underlying assumption was that children who had received this intervention for 4 to 6 months would have more advanced social and emotional behaviors and their attachment would be "stronger" as a consequence.

Based on the socialization scores of the Vineland Adaptive Behavior Scale (52), 7 children with autism (mean chronological age of 4 years) who were receiving the intervention were matched with 7 children who were not yet receiving the intervention. Attachment was measured using the Attachment Behavior Q-set, constructed by Waters and Deane (53) to yield an attachment score from 90 behavioral descriptive statements sorted based on extensive home observations of the child and caregiver.

The findings indeed indicated higher security scores for the treated children and higher maternal sensitivity scores for their mothers compared to the as-yet untreated children and their mothers. Interestingly, mothers of the treated children reported higher levels of stress compared to mothers of yet-untreated children, perhaps due to the intensity of the treatment and its lack of a specific module for the parents.

The Netherlands group also investigated the relation between parental sensitivity and child attachment (49). Parents of children with ASD were as sensitive as parents of children without ASD, but their children revealed more attachment disorganization and less child involvement. In the ASD group, more sensitive parents had more secure children, but this association was not found in the other groups.

Finally, Oppenheim and his colleagues examined how children's attachment classifications might associate with maternal insightfulness and resolution with the diagnosis status, as well as maternal sensitivity during mother-child interaction. Insightfulness refers to maternal ability to see the world from her child's point of view. Resolution with the diagnosis refers to the mother's ability to come to terms with the child's diagnosis and accept the child, with his/her strengths and vulnerabilities.

Oppenheim et al (42) found that mothers who were both insightful and resolved were more likely to have children with a secure attachment to them compared to mothers who were only insightful or only resolved or both non-insightful and non-resolved.

Eighty percent of the children of mothers who were both insightful and resolved had secure attachments, compared to 20% of the children whose mothers were either only insightful or only resolved and compared to 30% of the children whose mothers were neither insightful nor resolved. Further publications concerning this same sample (47, 54), reported that mothers of securely attached children with autism were more sensitive in their play interactions with their children compared to the mothers of insecurely attached children.

Moreover, maternal sensitivity as assessed during mother-child play interaction mediated between maternal representations (insightfulness and resolution) and children's attachment.

Conclusion

The studies on attachment in children with autism vary on many important dimensions, both from each other and from most studies conducted with young typically developing children. For one, in studies of attachment and autism, researchers often modified the Strange Situation Procedure (e.g., by using only one separation) and the original classification system and used behavioral frequencies rather than global classifications. The consequences of the variations in classification systems remain unknown. Furthermore, important demographic variables such as age, experience (e.g., types of early intervention, living arrangements), and mental age, as well as methodological differences regarding the employment of modifications in the strange situation and the utilization of various comparison groups hinder our ability to fully evaluate the findings of the various studies as whole. Finally, due to small sample sizes employed in the individual studies, it is still somewhat difficult to definitely reject the hypothesis that children with PDD have an increased risk for an insecure attachment relationship (33).

Yet, the field of attachment and autism deserves careful scrutiny in that secure attachment is a protective factor, whereas insecure attachment is a risk factor (55). As the current empirical review suggests, research thus far indicates that some and/or most children with autism are able to form secure attachments to their caregivers, even if we accept the claim proposed in the aforementioned meta-analysis from 2004 (35) that the frequency of such attachments is still somewhat lower in comparison to other groups.

Importantly, the one study in which mothers were interviewed about their perceptions regarding the attachment of their child with autism toward them (45) revealed that these mothers perceived their children as being less attached to them. Such parental perceptions of attachment are well studied in the typical population, so this is a gap in the literature which is now starting to be addressed (42, 47, 54). Of course, more studies regarding attachment are required with mothers as well as fathers. The association between maternal perceptions of their child's attachment toward them and the actual attachment of the children to their mothers also remains unknown at this time. Given the many difficulties that are faced by children with autism and their caregivers, it is reasonable to assume that parents and children could benefit from intervention programs that are based on attachment theory and research and that strive for optimal "good enough" parent-child relationships. Such intervention programs could target maternal representations (e.g., resolution with diagnosis) and behavior (e.g., emotional availability, sensitivity) and benefit the children and their families.

References

[1] Bowlby J. Attachment and loss: Vol. 1: New York: Basic Books, 1969.

[2] Ainsworth M, Bowlby J. An ethological approach to personality development. Am. Psychol. 1991;46:333-41.

[3] Bowlby J. The nature of the child's tie to the mother. Int. J. Psychoanal. 1958;39:1-24.

[4] Ainsworth M, Blehar M, Waters E, Wall S. Patterns of attachment: A psychological study of the strange situation. Hillsdale, NJ: Lawrence Erlbaum, 1978.

[5] Ainsworth M, Wittig B. Attachment and exploratory behavior of one-year-olds in a strange situation. In: Foss BM, ed. Determinants of infant behavior. London: Methuen, 1969:113-36.

[6] Connell J, Goldsmith H. A structural modeling approach to the study of attachment and strange situation behaviors. In: Emde RN, Harmon RJ, eds. The development of attachment and affiliative systems. New York: Plenum, 1982:213-43.

[7] Main M, Solomon J. Procedures for identifying disorganized/disoriented infants in the Ainsworth Strange Situation. In: Greenberg DC, Cummings EM, eds. Attachment in the preschool years: Theory, research, and intervention. Chicago: Univ. Chicago Press, 1990:121-60.

[8] Ainsworth M. Infant-mother attachment. Am Psychol 1979;34:932-7.

[9] Winnicott D. Ego distortion in terms of true and false self. The maturational processes and the facilitating environment: Studies in the theory of emotional development. New York: Int. Univ. Press, 1965:140-52.

[10] Van IJzendoorn M, Goldberg S, Kroonenberg P, Frenkel O. The relative effects of maternal and child problems on the quality of attachment: A meta-analysis of attachment in clinical samples. Child Dev. 1992;63:840-58.

[11] Main M. Cross-cultural studies of attachment organization: Recent studies, changing methodologies, and the concept of conditional strategies. Hum. Dev. 1990;33:48-61.

[12] van Ijzendoorn M, Schuengel C, Bakermans-Kranenburg M. Disorganized attachment in early childhood: Meta-analysis of precursors, concomitants, and sequelae. Dev. Psychopathol. 1999;11:225-50.

[13] Ainsworth M. Attachment: Retrospect and prospect. In: Parkes CM, Stevenson-Hinde J, eds. The place of attachment in human behavior. New York: Basic Books, 1982:3-30.

[14] Ainsworth M, Bell S, Stayton D, Schaffer H. The origins of human social relations. London: Acad. Press, 1971.

[15] Isabella R. Origins of attachment: Maternal interactive behavior across the first year. Child Dev. 1993;64:605-21.

[16] Belsky J, Garduque L, Hrncir E. Assessing performance, competence, and executive capacity in infant play: Relations to home environment and security of attachment. Dev. Psychol. 1984;20:406-17.

[17] Meins E, Fernyhough C, Russell J, Clark-Carter D. Security of attachment as a predictor of symbolic and mentalising abilities: A longitudinal study. Soc. Dev. 1998;7:1-24.

[18] Steele H, Steele M, Croft C, Fonagy P. Infant-mother attachment at one year predicts children's understanding of mixed emotions at six years. Soc. Dev. 1999;8:161-78.

[19] Fonagy P, Steele M, Steele H, Higgitt A, Target M. The theory and practice of resilience. J. Child Psychol. Psychiatr. 1994;35:231-57.

[20] Meins E. Security of attachment and the social development of cognition. Hove, UK: Psychol. Press, 1997.

[21] Bohlin G, Hagekull B, Rydell A. Attachment and social functioning: A longitudinal study from infancy to middle childhood. Soc. Dev. 2000;9:24-39.

[22] DeMulder E, Denham S, Schmidt M, Mitchell J. Q-sort assessment of attachment security during the preschool years: Links from home to school. Dev. Psychol. 2000;36:274-82.

[23] Park K, Waters E. Security of attachment and preschool friendships. Child Dev. 1989;60:1076-81.

[24] Sigman M, Ungerer J. Attachment behaviors in autistic children. J Autism Dev. Disord. 1984;14:231-44.

[25] Sigman M, Mundy P. Social attachments in autistic children. J. Am. Acad. Child Adolesc. Psychiatr. 1989;28:74-81.

[26] Capps L, Sigman M, Mundy P. Attachment security in children with autism. De.v Psychopathol. 1994;6:249-61.

[27] Shapiro T, Sherman M, Calamari G, Koch D. Attachment in autism and other developmental disorders. J. Am. Acad. Child Adolesc. Psychiatr. 1987;26:480-4.

[28] Rogers S, Ozonoff S, Maslin-Cole C. A comparative study of attachment behavior in young children with autism or other psychiatric disorders. J. Am. Acad. Child Adolesc. Psychiatr. 1991;30:483-8.

[29] Rogers S, Ozonoff S, Maslin-Cole C. Developmental aspects of attachment behavior in young children with pervasive developmental disorders. J. Am. Acad. Child Adolesc. Psychiatr. 1993;32:1274-82.

[30] Dissanayake C, Crossley S. Proximity and sociable behaviours in autism: Evidence for attachment. J. Child Psychol. Psychiatr. 1996;37:149-56.

[31] Dissanayake C, Crossley S. Autistic children's responses to separation and reunion with their mothers. J Autism Dev Disord 1997;27:295-312.

[32] Spencer AG. Attachment behaviors in children with autism. Diss. Abstr. Int. 1993;54:1321.

[33] Willemsen-Swinkels S, Bakermans-Kranenburg M, Buitelaar J, van IJzendoorn M, van Engeland H. Insecure and disorganised attachment in children with a pervasive developmental disorder: Relationship with social interaction and heart rate. J. Child Psychol. Psychiatr. Allied Disciplines 2000;41:759-67.

[34] Spangler G, Grossman K. Biobehavioral organization in securely and insecurely attached children. Child Dev. 1993;64:1439-50.

[35] Rutgers A, Bakermans-Kranenburg M, Ijzendoorn M, Berckelaer-Onnes I. Autism and attachment: A meta-analytic review. J. Child Psychol. Psychiatr. 2004;45:1123-34.

[36] Swinkels S, Dietz C, van Daalen E, Kerkhof I, van Engeland H, Buitelaar J. Screening for autistic spectrum in children aged 14 to 15 months. I: The development of the Early Screening of Autistic Traits Questionnaire (ESAT). J. Autism Dev. Disord 2006;36:723-32.

[37] Dietz C, Swinkels S, van Daalen E, van Engeland H, Buitelaar J. Screening for autistic spectrum disorder in children aged 14–15 months. II: population screening with the Early Screening of Autistic Traits Questionnaire (ESAT). Design and general findings. J. Autism Dev. Disord 2006;36:713-22.

[38] Naber F, Swinkels S, Buitelaar J, Bakermans-Kranenburg M, van IJzendoorn M, Dietz C, et al. Attachment in toddlers with autism and other developmental disorders. J. Autism Dev. Disord 2007;37:1123-38.

[39] Rutgers A, Van IJzendoorn M, Bakermans-Kranenburg M, Swinkels S. Autism and attachment: The attachment Q-sort. Autism 2007;11:187-200.

[40] Bakermans-Kranenburg M, Willemsen-Swinkels S, Van IJzendoorn M. Brief Attachment Screening Questionnaire. Leiden: Leiden Univ, Centre Child Fam. Stud., 2003.

[41] Waters E. QSTAT II. Computer scoring of the AQS. Stony Brook, NY: State Univ New York Stony Brook, Dept. Psychol., 1990.

[42] Oppenheim D, Koren-Karie N, Dolev S, Yirmiya N. Maternal insightfulness and resolution of the diagnosis are associated with secure attachment in preschoolers with Autism Spectrum Disorders. Child Dev. 2009;80:519-27.

[43] Taylor E, Target M, Charman T. Attachment in adults with high- functioning autism. Attach Hum. Dev. 2008;10:143-63.

[44] George C, Kaplan N, Main M. Adult attachment interview. Berkeley, CA: Univ Calif, 1985.

[45] Hoppes K, Harris S. Perceptions of child attachment and maternal gratification in mothers of children with autism and Down syndrome. J. Clin. Child Adolesc. Psychol. 1990;19:365-70.

[46] Marcu I, Oppenheim D, Koren-Karie N, Dolev S, Yirmiya N. Attachment and symbolic play in preschoolers with autism spectrum disorders. J. Autism Dev. Disord, In press.

[47] Koren-Karie N, Oppenheim D, Dolev S, Yirmiya N. Mothers of securely attached children with autism spectrum disorder are more sensitive than mothers of insecurely attached children. J. Child Psychol. Psychiatr. 2009;50:643-50.

[48] Rogers S, DiLALLA D. Age of symptom onset in young children with pervasive developmental disorders. J. Am. Acad. Child Adolesc. Psychiatr. 1990;29:863-72.

[49] van IJzendoorn M, Rutgers A, Bakermans-Kranenburg M, Swinkels S, van Daalen E, Dietz C, et al. Parental sensitivity and attachment in children with autism spectrum disorder: Comparison with children with mental retardation, with language delays, and with typical development. Child Dev. 2007;78:597-608.

[50] De Wolff M, van IJzendoorn M. Sensitivity and attachment: A meta-analysis on parental antecedents of infant attachment. Child Dev. 1997;68:571-91.

[51] Pechous E. Young children with autism and intensive behavioral programs: Effects on the primary attachment relationship. Diss Abstr. Int. Section B Sci. Engineering 2001;61:6145.
[52] Sparrow SS, Balla DA, Cicchetti DV. Vineland Adaptive Behavior Scales. Minneapolis: MN: Am. Guidance Serv., 1984.
[53] Waters E, Deane K. Defining and assessing individual differences in attachment relationships: Q-methodology and the organization of behavior in infancy and early childhood. Monogr. Soc. Res. Child Dev. 1985:41-65.
[54] Oppenheim D, Koren-Karie N, Dolev S, Yirmiya N. Maternal representations and child attachment in children with Autism Spectrum Disorder: The mediating role of maternal sensitivity. Attach Hum. Dev., in press.
[55] Yirmiya N. Attachment, development and quality of life. J. Child Psychol. Psychiatr. 2009;50:527-8.

In: Understanding Autism Spectrum Disorder
Editors: Ditza A Zachor and Joav Merrick
ISBN: 978-1-62081-353-9

Chapter 5

Compass: Finding direction for individuals with autism spectrum disorders

Lisa Ruble[1] **and Grace Mathai**[2]*
[1]Department of Educational, School, and Counseling Psychology, University of Kentucky, Lexington, Kentucky, US
[2]Department of Pediatrics, University of Louisville, Louisville, Kentucky, US

Abstract

Successfully meeting the unique behavioral health needs of individuals with autism spectrum disorders (ASD) is often a complex and daunting task for practitioners. Although evidence based practices are now available to facilitate decision-making and goal setting, few interventions have treatment protocols broad enough to span the diverse needs of children with ASD; those that do, rarely extend to outpatient, educational, or other community-based service settings.

Examples of community-based approaches that may help facilitate the development of personalized, socially valid and ecologically relevant treatment plans are necessary. The Collaborative Model for Promoting Competence and Success (COMPASS) is an ecological based, systematic, decision-making framework in which specialists work in collaboration with parents, caregivers, and other community-based practitioners and educators to a) identify socially valid and functional skills to teach, b) assess personal and environmental protective and risk factors that influence skill attainment and c) create personalized intervention plans based on effective teaching methods.

The purpose of this chapter is to describe the COMPASS protocol and apply the framework to two real-case scenarios of children with ASD referred to an outpatient clinic. One example focuses on a child who was referred for aggression; the second example highlights a child who was referred for social skills instruction.

* Correspondence: Lisa Ruble, Department of Educational, School and Counseling Psychology, University of Kentucky, 237 Dickey Hall, Lexington, KY 40506, United States. E-mail: lisa.ruble@uky.edu

Introduction

Effectively meeting the educational and behavioral health care needs of children, youth, and adults with autism spectrum disorder (ASD) remains a complex and overwhelming task for families and community based agencies responsible for services (1,2). The increased identification of children with autism (3) and subsequent growing number of parents and caregivers seeking services (1,4-6) creates a significant research to practice gap (7).

Programs responsible for care must be both accessible and effective. Descriptions of community-based treatment models that are not only broad enough to address the heterogeneous needs of individuals with ASD, but also sensitive enough to address the specific issues of individuals with ASD are lacking.

Research has shown that a 'one size fits all' approach to autism treatment has failed (7-9), and that more personalized interventions are necessary (10-12). Although attention to interventions in ASD has increased over the last several years (13), understanding which children benefit best by what approach remains unknown (9,13).

Another challenge is that the degree to which treatment research extends and translates to outpatient or community-based service settings has been questioned (14-16). Preliminary studies show promising results of time-limited (17,18) or community based interventions for young children (19-21).

The availability of treatment protocols that have demonstrated broad use within a clinic setting where youth and adults may seek services are lacking (16). Nevertheless, clinicians and practitioners are responsible for providing efficacious services to children, youth, and adults with ASD and must make attempts, themselves, to bridge the research-to-practice gap despite the lack of guidance from translational or effectiveness research (22). Often the case is that empirically supported interventions are modified by practitioners in ways that are feasible for everyday practice in outpatient settings (16,23).

The primary aim of this chapter is to describe a systematic decision-making and planning approach that helps address the need for more personalized interventions in ASD that can be administered within the outpatient clinical setting. The intervention planning framework focuses on a) intervention targets that are priorities to families and b) the identification of personal and environmental challenges and supports that can hinder or enhance goal attainment.

An assessment and treatment planning protocol called the Collaborative Model for Promoting Competence and Success (COMPASS) (24,25) that is based on contributions from ecological, developmental, and behavioral psychological perspectives is described. The approach has been tested in schools (26) and applied in outpatient clinics (27,28). In order to successfully implement the model, however, practitioners need to be knowledgeable of the underlying impairments in ASD as well as evidence based practices. Therefore, a brief review of theories of autism and empirically supported treatment methods is provided, followed by details on COMPASS.

Two case examples are presented that demonstrate both the social validity and the practical utility of the COMPASS model while upholding empirically sound practices within an outpatient treatment program. Although the case examples are based on children with ASD, the model lends itself to intervention goal setting and planning for youth and adults.

Personal challenges

Although individuals with ASD have primary challenges across several areas of development that result in failure or delayed development of critical skills, they also have unique learning styles (7) that are essential for practitioners to understand prior to treatment planning (16). In autism, failure in development begins to take notice in infancy when joint attention or the ability to coordinate attention with a social partner is disrupted (29). Inability in creating self-initiated episodes of joint attention is hypothesized to affect the input and richness of interactive experiences with others and cause interference in development that is thought to be associated with symptoms of autism.

Three cognitive theories offer important information for understanding the differences in social and cognitive thinking and unique learning styles associated with autism: a) theory of mind, b) weak central coherence and c) executive function (7,16,30). Each theory is important to understand because of the possible links that can be made to interventions commonly used for individuals with ASD. The first, theory of mind (TOM), is the ability to understand and attribute meaning of mental states of self and others (31). Difficulty understanding the sources of thoughts, feelings, and behaviors of self and others creates challenges in social problem solving and planful future interactions with others. The second, weak central coherence (WCC), refers to the tendency to focus on details rather than the overall meaning or global whole (32). Some have suggested that WCC could help explain problems individuals with ASD have in generalizing information from one situation to another (33). The last theory, executive function (EF), is a general term that refers to the abilities to initiate, sustain, shift, and inhibit behavior (34). EF problems can be attributed to difficulties taking in multiple types of information, making decisions quickly based on this information, and evaluating the outcomes of the situation.

Debate ensues over the universality, specificity, and uniqueness of these three theories with regard to autism, and arguments can be made on the overlap or primacy of the theories (30). Nevertheless, they offer helpful frameworks for characterizing many of the personal challenges associated with ASD, and more importantly, planning for interventions. Understanding how these theories can lend themselves to possible corresponding strategies (i.e., environmental supports) that can help compensate for the challenges (7) is essential. If only a behavioral approach is taken for intervention planning, important information that can be associated with cognitive influences goes undetected, resulting in insufficient and ineffective treatment plans (16). Clinicians who are able to understand the relationships between the underlying and accumulative effects of disordered theory of mind, executive function, and central coherence and behavioral symptoms are better prepared to create, adapt, apply, evaluate, and monitor psychosocial interventions for individuals with ASD (16).

Empirically supported interventions

Empirically supported interventions include comprehensive approaches that target the core impairments in autism (13,35) or specific teaching methods that focus on acquisition of new or discrete skill sets (e.g.,(36)). Examples of comprehensive programs are the Denver Model (37), Intensive Behavioral Intervention (38), and TEACCH (10). Several sources are available that summarize these and other examples of comprehensive programs and evidence based practices (9,11,13).

Empirically supported intervention methods designed to teach targeted skills are based on single or combined theoretical frameworks such as learning or behavioral theories (e.g.,(39)), developmental frameworks (e.g.,(12)), and social cognitive models (e.g.,(40)). The most studied method is the behavioral model (13). Applied behavior analysis (ABA) is useful for reducing aberrant behaviors, increasing desirable behaviors, and teaching new skills (36). ABA is an operant behavioral approach that targets child responsivity to prompts and cues. Extensive data collection and ongoing monitoring of measured progress are essential elements. Measurement is often based on frequency counts of isolated behaviors. ABA is an umbrella term that can include different methods such as discrete trial training, and more contemporary approaches of incidental teaching (41) and pivotal response training (42) designed to address limitations of discrete trial training (35).

Developmental approaches are child-directed and emphasize child initiation as the primary outcome. Multiple intervention targets are emphasized during a particular activity. Measurement approaches such as videotaping and time sampling are used to free up the adult to engage with the child rather than focus mainly on data collection (12) during teaching interactions.

A third notable approach important for children with autism is structured teaching (10,43). Structured teaching is a departure from the other two predominant paradigms because the methodology incorporates cognitive social learning theory into intervention assessment, planning, and teaching. It is also based on the cognitive strengths and challenges of persons with ASD, and takes into account the role of cognitive influence on behavior.

In their final conclusions of their review of evidence based practices in autism, Rogers and Vismara (14) state that despite a limited number of published randomized controlled studies in early intervention (e.g.,(44-48)), general results are that as a group, children with autism benefit from interventions that are specialized to their focused needs. They remind readers of the lack of comparative research, and thus, inability to state whether one treatment method is better than another.

There now appears to be a growing consensus and general agreement that one treatment method is inappropriate for all children or for all skills to be taught. Teaching a child to initiate will be more challenging when using an adult-directed responsive-focused intervention compared to a child-directed teaching approach; conversely, selecting a child-directed initiation-focused approach to teach a child to complete a novel task from start to finish is incongruous with the aims of the teaching outcome, and thus, an adult initiated discrete trial and / or structured teaching approach makes more sense. It is possible that each of the distinct methodologies based on behavioral, developmental, or social cognitive approaches, when combined in a systematic fashion, may produce the best child outcomes. However, due to a lack of research, it is not known if an integrated approach using systematic, comprehensive, and intensive methods is better than a single treatment method approach. It stands to reason, though, that the selection of teaching methods when matched with both (a) the skill that is targeted for teaching and (b) the specific learning profile based on child strengths and challenges provides a unique opportunity for the development of exceptionally personalized intervention plans.

Compass model

Given the necessity to consider the child's personal strengths and challenges as well as the environment in which the child learns and lives, a systematic decision-making and collaborative planning process is described. The Collaborative Model for Promoting Competence and Success (COMPASS) (25, 26) is a comprehensive planning approach that allows for the inclusion of the efficacious techniques described above. In this decision-making model, practitioners work in collaboration with parents and caregivers to identify socially valid and important skills to teach. Challenges to learning, such as personal and environmental risk factors, as well as the essential personal and environmental supports required for achievement and learning are reviewed (see figure 1). Personal risk factors refer to the difficulties inherent to the characteristics of autism and set the stage for learning challenges, whereas environmental risk factors are those that inhibit success and may be more amenable to direct change (e.g. parents who may lack sufficient understanding of autism, lack of alternative communication methods, lack of routines, etc.).

Conversely, supports are characterized as personal strengths and preferences of individuals with autism, and as environmental modifications and adaptations to compensate for challenges and risk factors. Numerous studies have lent support to the favorable impact that appropriate personal and environmental supports provide (e.g., (49-51)).

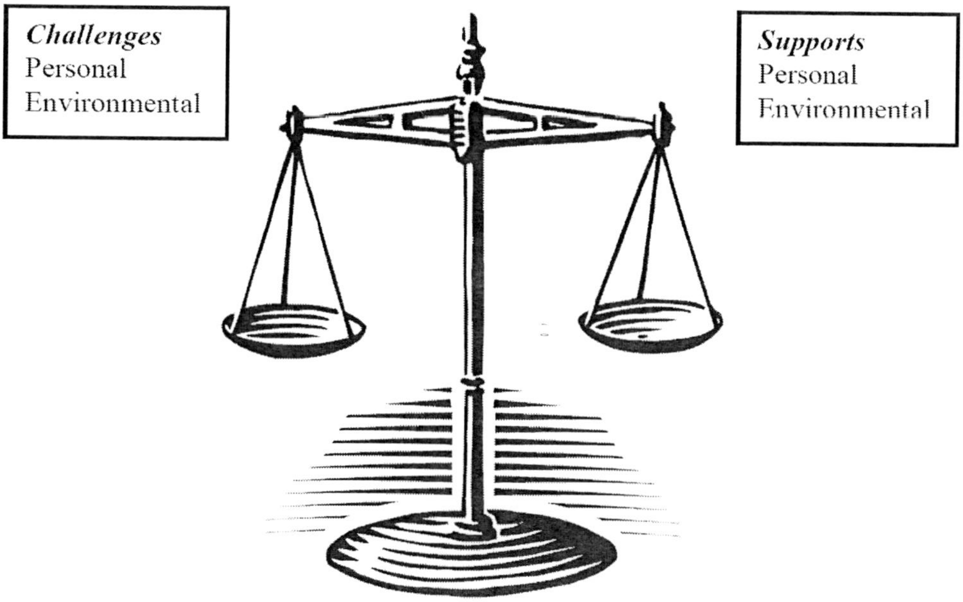

Figure 1. COMPASS Model.

The COMPASS model incorporates these factors with behavioral, cognitive, developmental, and social learning techniques to enhance the skills of both children and those living or working with them (e.g., caregivers and teachers). Two case examples are provided. Both examples are based on real concerns presented by children seen in an outpatient medical setting.

Case story one (Karl)

Background. Karl was a 9 year old boy who was diagnosed with autism at the age of three years by an experienced developmental behavioral pediatrician. At the time of the evaluation in 2006, Karl had non verbal (pragmatic) language deficits, his vocabulary score was below an age equivalent of 6 years 2 months. His full scale IQ on the Wechsler Abbreviated Scale of Intelligence was 83 (13th percentile); a nonverbal IQ score using the Test of Nonverbal Intelligence, Third Edition (TONI-3), revealed a quotient of 97 (42nd percentile). His parents brought him to the university-based outpatient autism intervention program with a number of concerns related to behavioral and social difficulties.

Assessment. The COMPASS (25) framework served as the initial organizing approach. Karl's parents were informed that the purpose of COMPASS was to assist in the identification of interpersonal strengths and weaknesses as well as environmental supports and challenges that compound or impact upon Karl's ability to be resilient in his environment. The assessment revealed the following information in table 1.

Table 1. Karl's COMPASS Assessment

Personal Challenges	*Personal Supports*
• Behavioral • Impulsive • Low frustration tolerance • Perfectionistic tendencies • Unusual mannerisms such as hand flapping *Social* • Problems initiating and maintaining interactions • Problems with perspective taking • Low social reciprocity *Emotional* • Worries over many things, currently thunderstorms and tornadoes. • Inability to expressing worries appropriately *Sensory* • Problems with being overwhelmed by sounds/crowds	• Is good at sciences and math • Likes video games, animals and going on adventures. • Affectionate • Wants to hang out with peers and have friends • Very observant • Likes to do chores and help • Motivated to have important roles such as "helper" • Visual learner • Likes to draw
Environmental Challenges • Lack of appropriate services • Lack of supportive peers • Environments with a lot of extraneous stimuli such as lights, sounds and crowds • Thunderstorms and tornadoes or threats of storms	*Environmental Supports* • Speech language services in school • Behavior intervention in school • Parents as strong advocates

Information revealed a number of personal challenges, many characteristic of children with autism, but also a number of personal strengths. Most notable was Karl's desire to make friends with other children as well as please others. In addition, important environmental challenges were also identified that included a lack of a supportive peer group and trained personnel at his school. To help counterbalance these challenges, environmental supports revealed that his parents are strong advocates that with knowledge and training, could transfer information and skills taught during the therapy sessions to the school setting. It was clear that in order for this to happen, a generalization plan was essential.

Background information

Parent/Teacher priorities. Karl's mom reported that her major concerns were Karl's personal challenges in initiating with others appropriately and maintaining reciprocal interactions. He often holds back and plays alongside his peers because he does not know how to approach them and ask to join in play. She was becoming increasingly worried about his social isolation and lack of friendships. A second concern was his increasing fear of thunderstorms and tornadoes. Initially Karl would express worry and fear when a tornado siren went off, running off to the basement and hiding; now he was doing the same behavior if he thought a thunderstorm was approaching or observed clouds darkening the sky. These behaviors were often disruptive in school and at home. He had stopped accompanying the family to parks or other recreational activities for fear that a thunderstorm may befall them.

His teacher reported that Karl has trouble working in groups and engaging with his peers. He was often observed to play alongside his peers. She also expressed concerns regarding Karl's perfectionistic tendencies. Overall, both Karl's parent and teacher agreed that their concerns were Karl's social interaction skills with peers and worries and preoccupations with the weather.

Child assessment

Assessment of social skills: Because the primary concerns focused on social issues, the TRIAD social skills assessment (52) was administered to help identify specific social targets for intervention. The assessment is a criterion-referenced evaluation of three major components of social skills: a) affective understanding and expression of emotions, b) cognitive understanding of perspective taking and problem solving skills and c) behavioral skills of initiating, maintaining and terminating interactions as well as responding to the social bids from others.

Affective understanding and perspective taking: Karl was shown several pictures of children's faces and given various pictorial scenarios that contained a problem involving two or more children. When shown the pictures, Karl was able to accurately identify the emotions on the children's faces and relate a time when he might have experienced the emotion. When asked what would make a significant other (i.e., a specific family member) experience the similar emotion, responses were often "I don't know." When shown pictures of problem situations, Karl was able to identify the problems, but had difficulty generating plausible solutions to solve the problems. Overall, he displayed challenges in taking another's perspective and generating ideas to solve social problems..

Preferred activities: To obtain information on Karl's social motivation (i.e., interest in interacting with other children), Karl was presented a list of activities and then asked to rate his preference in performing preferred activities with friends vs. family vs. by himself. This task involved presenting Karl with a worksheet of a list of "things to do" and "places to go" and asking him to rate how much he likes each one by circling a number that corresponded to a scale (i.e., not at all; a little; a lot). Overall, Karl reported he liked to play on a playground, play video games, play on the computer, play with toys, build things with legos or blocks, draw or paint pictures, cook or bake, and watch television or videos very much. Of these activities, he preferred to do most alone, except for playing on the playground and building things with legos and blocks, which he indicated a preference for doing with other kids. Overall, Karl appeared to be hesitant to be involved with other kids while completing preferred activities. But activities that would keep Karl's interest were identified and could be used as environmental supports.

Role play skills: Karl's ability to understand and perform role-plays was assessed. He was asked to interact with the examiner in role plays that dealt with possible daily situations. During the role plays, Karl demonstrated difficulties initiating appropriately. For example, he often avoided greetings and started a conversation with a direct request or comment that he had on his mind. Very soon into the role-play conversation, Karl terminated the interaction and requested to go to the toilet. He conversed with a monotone voice quality and facial expressions were restricted; eye contact was diminished during the entire interaction.

Treatment goals: The COMPASS and Triad Social Skills Assessment revealed and clarified two major areas of concern: a) initiating appropriately and maintaining reciprocal interactions with peers and adults and b) managing his anxiety regarding the weather without interruption of daily activities. These two goals were targeted in a treatment plan.

Treatment plan

Initiating appropriately and maintaining reciprocal interactions with peers and adults: Initiating with others involves several types of skills. For Karl's therapy plan, initiating a variety of requests with peers, giving complements, and having conversations were taught. For each of these skills, a four step procedure was used to develop the components of the intervention plan (see Table 2;16,23). First, a Social Story™ (53-55) was used to introduce the importance of the skill from another's perspective and address Karl's personal challenges in theory of mind and weak central coherence that might be related to understanding and teaching the skill. Social Stories™ provide written information that describes situations, other's perspectives about the situation, skill, and responses, and why the skill is relevant to Karl. Next, other activities were implemented that tapped into Karl's relative strength in visual vs auditory learning. First, an activity that depicts the positive skill in a concrete and visual manner was introduced. Often this is a sorting activity that breaks down the skill into its component parts. Also depicted is the correct vs. incorrect way to perform the skill; the use of picture cards (e.g., pictures from magazines, hand drawings on 3x5 cards) helps children develop a concrete depiction of the positive skill being taught (56). Third, role-plays were used to practice the skill and show a visual model of the skill. Actual situations that the child has encountered are used as part of the role-plays as much as possible. This information typically comes from parents and family members. Fourth, homework was provided to enhance the likelihood that the skill would generalize to settings outside the clinic. If parents, caregivers, or significant others are not part of the treatment session, either through observation or as part of family therapy, it is necessary that as much information as possible be shared with them. Due to the significant issues in individuals with ASD generalizing information from one context to another, it is necessary that plans for generalization such as homework and family communication about the session be in place.

For Karl, the first step of applying a social story for facilitating his understanding of the importance of initiating with other children focused specifically on initiating to give a greeting, join peers, and ask for help so that he could begin to have more friends. The concept of "social circles" was used to identify different people he encounters and the appropriate greetings that correspond to this person. Karl matched scripts of examples of specific types of greetings provided on 3x5 cards to a list of a variety of adults and peers he knew in his environment (e.g., classmates, parents, other family members, grocery clerk, teachers, neighbors, postman). Other scripts that could be used for initiating in a number of different contexts were also generated and taught, such as asking to join classmates at play, asking another classmate to join in play, offering to share toys or snacks, and offering to help. Visuals depicting the appropriate body language to use were taught to emphasize eye contact, facial expressions, posture and proximity to others. Special attention was given regarding Karl's voice intonation. The right way to initiate vs. the wrong way to initiate was also modeled for Karl. After observing the role-play, he then identified the characteristics that make up good initiations and described why this had a better consequence than examples of poor initiations. The Social Skills Picture book (57) was an excellent resource that was used to give Karl step-by-step instructions on how to successfully initiate within different contexts. Several opportunities to practice using role plays with a therapist and then peers within a group setting gave him more confidence to practice in real world settings. Each role play was followed by feedback. Different scenarios were also modeled for Karl when an attempt to initiate to play with another peer was rejected, such as asking another child to play and the child refused.

Karl was also taught to compliment others. Emphasis was placed on focusing on the "other." He also was taught the various types of compliments he could pay others regarding their appearance, their personality, or how they do things. Various examples were demonstrated to Karl regarding these different compliments. Karl practiced complimenting with the therapist, and completed homework for practice in other settings. Naturally occurring reinforcers, such as his mom's responses to his compliments, further strengthened his resolve to compliment his peers in his neighborhood. Sorting compliments into categories were used to teach the difference between warm messages (compliments) or cold messages (insensitive/mean comments).

Karl was then taught how to have a conversation once he could join a group of peers at play. First, he was taught to approach them, wait for a pause, get their attention, give them a compliment or a warm message and then ask to join in play. Role plays used with Karl to teach the different steps, as well as how he could respond to different responses from his peers, such as when he was refused. Karl understood that refusals from peers were okay, and that they did not mean that he was disliked; he just had to keep trying. Karl was taught to show interest in other's topics or objects of interest and encouraged to ask appropriate "Wh" questions or make appropriate comments to further the interaction. He was also taught the two question rule, (58). This rule emphasized "asking the same question back." If someone asked Karl about his weekend, he could respond to the question and then ask the same question back. Visuals and modeling was used to demonstrate to Karl what active listening looked like, which involved making eye contact, nodding, asking questions and making comments while the other person was speaking.

All 12 therapy sessions were observed by Karl's parents. Verbal praise and other material rewards were used to encourage appropriate responses and modeled for his parents. They played a major role in helping Karl carry over his treatment plan to naturalistic settings, giving him opportunities to practice in real life settings and making sure his teachers were aware of the strategies in place so they could help implement them and reinforce accordingly at school.

Table 2. Four step procedure for skills teaching

1. Define the skill and explain why it is important
2. Demonstrate what the skill looks like (the right way vs the wrong way)
3. Perform role plays demonstrating the skill
4. Provide homework to practice the skill

Managing anxiety and avoidance. The second area of focus for Karl involved coping with his fears. A cognitive behavioral treatment approach (CBT) was used with Karl to decrease his anxiety and increase social participation in outdoor activities and with his family. The CBT protocol based on Kendall (59) was used which provided a general framework for Karl's treatment; however, strategies from other authors were also incorporated into the treatment package (60). Specific modifications were made to the treatment outline to make it more applicable for children with autism, using the four-step procedure outlines in table 2. However, due to the cognitive aspects of his fear of thunderstorms, the first several activities focused on identifying cognitive attributions and competing responses (helpful cognitions, relaxation strategies, and use of systematic relaxation).

To accomplish these goals, the first step involved using a social story to help Karl develop an awareness of his anxiety and the consequences of it on himself (his behaviors and his emotions) and others. A sorting task was used to help Karl identify his environmental triggers, his physical (internal) responses, his cognitions, and his behavioral (observable) responses. Karl was quite artistic and began to draw his fears/environmental triggers. He began to label these triggers as "monsters" who were trying to fight him. He was quite resolute in that he did not want to be a "scaredy cat" but wanted to be a "cool guy" and was determined to fight these fear monsters. Karl was then taught a relaxation technique involving progressive muscle relaxation and visual imagery. Initially he required prompting to practice followed by tangible reward or praise. He learned to practice this technique on a daily basis and found that relaxing his body calmed him down. The next step involved teaching Karl to discriminate between his "Helpful" thoughts and his "Unhelpful" thoughts. Thoughts that expected bad things to happen when a storm was on its way versus thoughts that helped him calm down and expected him to be safe were listed. He was taught to challenge the unhelpful thoughts and replace them with helpful ones instead that would lead to more success and most importantly for Karl, be a "cool guy." Karl even drew the weapons he would use to tackle his "worry monsters."

Next, Karl created a stress hierarchy using a visual stress thermometer (61; Figure 2).

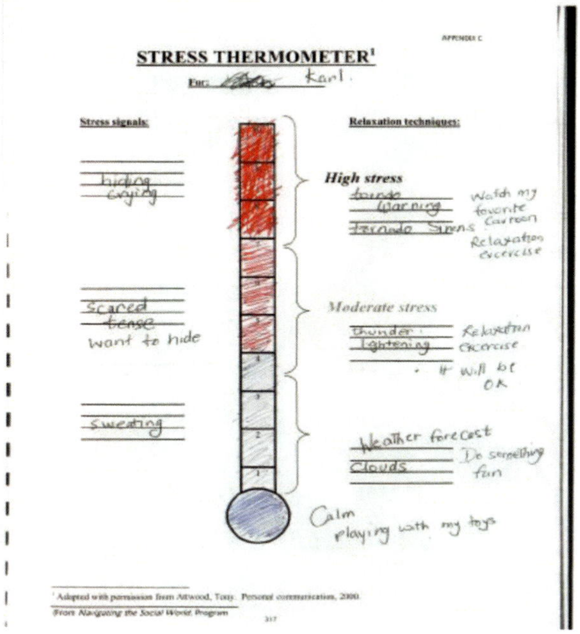

Figure 2. Stress Thermometer.

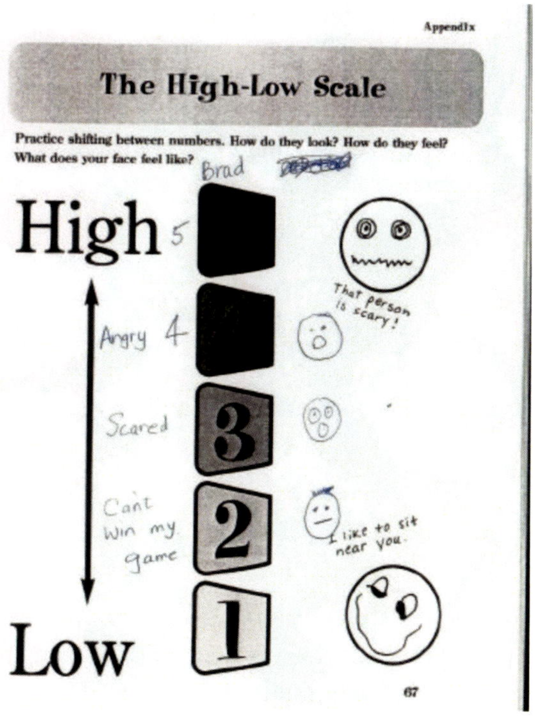

Figure 3. Emotion Scale.

He identified those activities that helped him be calm, such as art, and then he gradually identified stressful events that evolved into fear and avoidance. The lowest item (and most stressful) involved forecast of bad weather, followed by thunder clouds, heavy rain, thunder, lightening and so on. Parent interview also confirmed the order on the stress hierarchy. This set the stage for graduated exposure and parent training.

Karl's parents were counseled on how to respond to Karl's preoccupations and obsessions of the weather by reassuring him once and then redirecting him to the task. They had a specific 15 minute time period once a day called "worry time" to address his fears.

Parents encouraged Karl to participate in activities involving the outdoors even when there was a forecast of rain. These activities were always paired with highly reinforcing items or activities for Karl, such as eating his favorite snacks on the trip and being chosen as mom's special "helper" with assisting his little brother.

After the rain, he was encouraged to play in the puddles with his little brother. Karl was reinforced and praised every time he participated on an item identified on his stress thermometer (see Figure 2).

Six month follow up

Goal attainment scaling (GAS; 62) was used to track Karl's progress. GAS is based on a 5-point scale ranging from -2 to + 2. Current symptoms and presenting concerns are rated at zero, a worsening of symptoms receive a progressive negative score downward to -2 and improvements get a positive score up to +2. After 12, 60-minute therapy session, Karl's parents rated his ability to initiate and have reciprocal interactions with his peers at a +1, indicating much improvement by almost 50% in terms of frequency of initiating and interacting in a reciprocal manner. Likewise improvements were also observed by his teacher. A rating of +2 was obtained on his ability to handle his anxiety regarding storms and ability to continue daily activities in an uninterrupted manner. However, he had developed some fears around hand sanitizers, insisting at school to use soap and water to wash his hands when the sanitizer was available. Parents were using the same strategies to help Karl overcome this anxiety as they had regarding storms.

Case story two (Brad)

Brad was a 10-year old male with a diagnosis of autism received at age 7 years from a licensed clinical psychologist of a local area pediatric clinic. He presented with a number of behavioral and social difficulties. A review of previous assessments indicated that Brad's expressive and receptive language skills were in the mild to moderate range of impairment, and his cognitive abilities as assessed on the Kaufman Brief Intelligence Test-II resulted in an IQ composite of 75 which is below average according to the Kaufman classification system. Brad was able to express his needs and wants in single words and phrases, and was often difficult to understand due to his articulation difficulties. His adaptive abilities as measured on the Vineland Adaptive behavior Scales indicated low to moderately low functioning in the communication, daily living, socialization and motor domains.

Assessment

The ecological and whole-child approach to assessment was once again applied using the COMPASS framework. A summary of Brad's personal and environmental supports and challenges revealed the following in table 3. While several personal challenges were identified, it was also revealed that Brad had many strengths to be included in a treatment plan. He understands work-reward routines, wants to please others, and likes to earn rewards. Also revealed were notable environmental challenges that would need to be considered in a treatment plan.

Environmental challenges included a lack of routine and structure at home, unlimited access to preferred items (that could be used a rewards for positive behavior), and changes in home routines due to his father being away on military leave. Environmental supports that were in place at the time of the assessment were involvement of a behavior specialist, school support through an Individual Education plan, and his mother's pursuit of additional support for herself and her son. Identification of these environmental supports indicated that plans for collaboration with the behavior specialist who is working with Brad at school be included in his treatment plan as well as discussion with his mother about her own coping strategies and ways to enhance her support and sense of parental competency.

Table 3. Brad's COMPASS Assessment

Personal Challenges	*Personal Supports*
• Low frustration tolerance • Expressive and receptive language difficulties • Problems listening and following directions • Problems transitioning from one activity to the next • Restricted interests • Soils self • Inability to self soothe	• Understands concept of working for a reward • Understands concept of finished • Likes to play with other children • Likes to play videogames • Likes to earn rewards and praise • Can be affectionate • Strong visual learning skills (compared to receptive language or listening skills)
Environmental Challenges	*Environmental Supports*
• Single parent since dad is outside the country on military duty • Lack of structure in the home environment • Unrestrained access to play materials.	• A therapist working on behavioral difficulties • Mom who is seeking help for self and Brad and is attending a support group • An Individualized Education Plan (IEP) and receives speech language services at school

Presenting concerns

Brad's mom was mainly concerned about tantrums and aggression that consisted of Brad throwing himself on the floor, destroying property, and hitting others.

She was concerned about his safety and the safety of her other children at home during these episodes. Tantrums lasted from 15 to 20 minutes, and left both Brad and mom exhausted. She was also concerned about Brad soiling himself on a regular basis. He had both urinary and bowel accidents, although he had been fully toilet trained by age five. Consults with the pediatrician did not indicate any medical causes of the problem.

Brad's teacher, on the other hand, reported concerns about Brad's difficulties with transitioning from one activity to the next, especially when it involved transitions from a preferred activity to a nonpreferred activity. Bowel and urinary accidents also took place in school.

Child assessment

The child assessment consisted of a semi-structured, interactive, activity-based evaluation of several aspects of social and communication development that included how well Brad initiated and responded to social bids, took turns, and made requests. With regard to Brad's communication, he spoke in short sentences and simple phrases. He was often difficult to understand due to his articulation difficulties. As soon as work tasks were presented (e.g., puzzles), Brad began to protest, saying "No", and pushed the materials away; however, when he was shown a visual prompt demonstrating "first work" then "reward," he became more compliant. Brad followed directives and transitioned through a series of activities using a visual picture schedule and the work and reward prompt. When presented with an activity designed to elicit requesting (e.g., during a puzzle activity, a piece of the puzzle is withheld by the examiner), he did not ask directly for the missing piece, but looked concerned and mentioned the name of the piece. He responded to questions, but was unable to have a reciprocal conversation or initiate conversation. Brad was observed to use trial and error to arrive at right solutions, he demonstrated understanding of the concept of "finished" and "working for a reward'. He did have difficulty with waiting and became whiny when awaiting his turn to play.

Due to parental concerns focusing primarily on noncompliance and aggression, a functional assessment of the problematic behaviors was conducted (63). Over a two-week time period, Brad's mom and teacher recorded the frequency of each of three identified problematic behaviors (soiling, tantrumming, and noncompliance with transitions) and times during the day when these behaviors occurred. His mom and teacher also recorded the antecedents (what happened before the behavior) and consequences (what happened after the behavior or how the behavior was responded to). From this descriptive behavior analysis, the following information was determined and is listed in Table 4.

Brad's mother reported that soiling and tantrumming occurred about equally each day (one to three times) and problems transitioning more frequently, about three to five times daily. Analysis of possible functions of the behaviors indicated that soiling may be related to transitions and not wanting to stop a preferred activity. Tantrums often occurred when told no or restricted from a desired activity.

Even though problems transitioning occurred more frequently at home and at school, it was important for Brad's mom to address the other behaviors first, and she identified tantrums and soiling as her major concerns she wanted to be addressed immediately.

To begin, a specific behavioral objective was identified for tantrumming: Brad will comply with directives and respond to "no" appropriately with a 50 % decrease in tantrumming behavior (and 50% increase in compliance).

Table 4. Analysis of Brad's Behavior

Behavior	Frequency	What might the behavior communicate?
Soiling (urinary/bowel accidents)	About 1 to 3 times a day both at home and at school, more frequently at home than at school	Tends to occur when Brad is too involved or preoccupied with his games or activities of high interest. Indicates difficulty halting or terminating an activity to take a bathroom break.
Tantrums (hitting others, destroying of property, screaming)	About 1 to 3 times a day; mostly at home	Most often tends to occur when a demand is placed on him; when he is told "no" or is asked to "wait."
Noncompliance with transitions (whining, saying no, pulling away)	3 to 5 times a day; both at home and in school	Tends to occur when Brad is asked to terminate an existing activity and move on to the next activity, especially if he is transitioning to a less preferred activity.

After the objective was established, a collaborative teaching plan was developed with input from the other behavior therapist that he was seeing as well as from Brad's mother.

Intervention plan

The comprehensive intervention plan involved several components and, like Karl's plan, was based on a cognitive behavioral framework (64). It included a didactic component that addressed Brad's comprehension of his emotions and how to express them appropriately using a number of positive behavior supports including visuals and social stories. It included a differential reinforcement strategy that specifically acknowledged positive alternatives to the negative behavior, thereby enhancing and strengthening desired behaviors. Finally a generalization plan from the clinical environment into Brad's home and school environments was created and implemented. Parent support through training from modeling, corrective feedback, and rehearsal was provided to help with generalization.

To address his understanding of the problem behaviors, a social story was introduced, delineating the essentials of why it was important to stay calm and how to respond when frustrated or upset, by asking for a break, asking for help or using a strategy to calm down (e.g., breathing and counting). Visuals were created that prompted him to request these alternatives, such as an "I want break" card and a "I need help" card. He was taught to use a 5- point scale (65) visual to help him understand how his emotions could escalate from being calm to losing control. The visual also addressed the environmental triggers, body responses and associated "angry" thoughts. Sorting activities were used to enhance his awareness of these different triggers that contributed to his behaviors. Brad was also taught a relaxation strategy, to breathe and count using a "count down" visual that was created by the therapist and involved a laminated card with numbers one to 10 and finally asking "Am I calm?"

The next step involved teaching Brad how to use these supports effectively within the clinic setting.

The assessment had indicated that Brad had worked well transitioning through different activities using a visual schedule. Similar schedules were created using pictures from software programs such as Mayer-Johnson's Board-maker software or online from Google images.

The schedule indicated when certain activities would take place and what would come next giving Brad a certain predictability about the activities of the day as well as highlighting how much work needed to be done before reinforcement (i.e., play) could occur.

During tasks that were difficult, an "I need help" visual was strategically positioned on his desk that prompted him to ask for help rather than getting frustrated and having a tantrum. Soon a choice board was created that had visuals that could prompt him to "wait', "take turns," "ask for a break," or "ask for help." Every time Brad used these visuals, he was reinforced and praised for his appropriate behaviors.

Play activities that involved turn taking and waiting (to help him manage frustration) were used to teach Brad to learn to wait for his turn while playing a game or awaiting his turn to play with a favorite toy. A reward system was introduced that involved a system of earning tokens. Each 50-minute therapy session was divided into five segments and at the end of each segment, Brad was asked to self monitor his behavior with regard to listening and staying calm. If he correctly indicated that he has been doing both positive behaviors, he earned a token. After he had earned five tokens, he could exchange the tokens for a reward.

Next came the generalization component. Brad's mom had been observing each session through a one-way mirror in the clinic. Once Brad had learned to use the supports effectively with the therapist, his mother was encouraged to use them with Brad during the session.

A second set of visuals were created for mom to use at home. Practice during sessions with the therapist enabled her to use the visuals and reinforcement systems with slight adaptations for home. His mom also shared the teaching plan with Brad's teacher and behavior therapist. Visual schedules were incorporated during his day at school to facilitate transitions.

The second concern around toileting accidents was addressed through use of a visual schedule that incorporated toilet breaks on an hourly basis. At home, where these accidents mostly occurred, a timer was set to prompt Brad to use the toilet on an hourly basis. Brad was not allowed to continue with the activity unless he had taken the toilet break as indicated by the timer. This required supervision from mom initially; she was taught to use a firm, clear directive. If this directive was not followed, then she would withdraw the activity from Brad until the directive was followed. She was also instructed to state the directive in the positive, remain calm, and ignore his tantrumming. As soon as he had followed the directive, he could be rewarded with being able to resume his activity.

Brad's mom also was instructed that as soon as the behavior plan was implemented, she could expect some worsening of his behaviors and was advised to continue with the plan despite the exacerbations.

Six month follow up

At the end of six months and the completion of eight 60-minute therapy sessions, GAS was used to determine Brad's progress. Mom rated his tantrumming behaviors at a +1 (from a scale of -2 to +2). Tantrums still occurred, but with about 70% less frequency and intensity compared to baseline.

With regard to his toileting behaviors, she rated him with a +2 as there were no further incidents of soiling once the intervention plan had been implemented.

Conclusion

In conclusion, both case studies represent a comprehensive approach to assessment and treatment planning. A thorough understanding of the child's strengths and challenges within the broader ecological framework of COMPASS provides the essential ingredients in conceptualizing a socially valid and personalized treatment plan. Changes in behavior cannot occur in isolation.

Concurrent with teaching, skill building, and use of necessary behavior supports is also the *process* by which environments are created that are conducive in sustaining and fortifying the strengths of children and families.

References

[1] Ruble LA, Heflinger CA, Renfrew JW, Saunders RC. Access and service use by children with autism spectrum disorders in Medicaid Managed Care. J. Autism Dev. Disord. 2005;35(1):3-13.

[2] Stahmer AC. The basic structure of community early intervention programs for children with autism: provider descriptions. J. Autism Dev. Disord. 2007;37(7):1344-54.

[3] Yeargin Allsopp M, Rice C, Karapurkar T, Doernberg N, Boyle C, and Murphy C. Prevalence of autism in a US metropolitan area. JAMA: J. Am. Med. Assoc. 2003;289(1): 49-55.

[4] Cassidy A, McConkey R, Truesdale-Kennedy M, Slevin E. Preschoolers with autism spectrum disorders: The impact on families and the supports available to them. Early Child Dev. Care 2008; 178(2):115-28.

[5] Krauss MW, Gulley S, Sciegaj M, Wells N. Access to specialty medical care for children with mental retardation, autism, and other special health care needs. Ment. Retard 2003;41(5):329-39.

[6] Symon JB. Parent Education for Autism: Issues in providing services at a distance. J. Pos. Beh. Interv. 2001;3(3):160.

[7] Volkmar FR, Lord C, Bailey A, Schultz RT, Klin A. Autism and pervasive developmental disorders. J. Child Psychol. Psychiatry 2004; 45(1):135-70.

[8] Kasari C. Assessing change in early intervention programs for children with autism. J. Autism Dev. Disord. 2002;32(5):447-61.

[9] Simpson RL. Evidence-based practices and students with autism spectrum disorders. Focus Autism Other Dev Disabl 2005;20(3): 140-9.

[10] Mesibov G, Shea V, Schopler E. The TEACCH Approach to Autism Spectrum Disorders. New York: Springer, 2006.

[11] Odom SL, Brown WH, Frey T, Karasu N, Smith-Canter LL, Strain P S. Evidence-based practices for young children with autism: contributions for single-subject design research. Focus Autism and Other Dev Disabl 2003;18(3):166-75.

[12] Prizant BM, Wetherby AM, Rydell, PJ. Communication intervention issues for children with autism spectrum disorders. Baltimore, MD: Paul H Brookes, 2000.

[13] Rogers SJ, and Vismara LA. Evidence-based comprehensive treatments for early autism. J. Clin. Child Adolesc. Psychol. 2008;37(1):8-38.

[14] Anan RM, Warner LJ, McGillivary JE, Chong IM, Hines S J. Group Intensive Family Training (GIFT) for preschoolers with autism spectrum disorders. Behav. Intervent. 2008;23(3):165-80.
[15] Perrin CJ, Perrin SH, Hill EA, DiNovi K. Brief functional analysis and treatment of elopement in preschoolers with autism. Behav. Intervent. 2008; 23(2):87-98.
[16] Ruble L, Willis H, Crabtree VM. Social skills group therapy for autism spectrum disorders. Clin. Case. Stud. 2008;7(4): 287-300.
[17] Vismara LA, Colombi C, Rogers SJ. Can one hour per week of therapy lead to lasting changes in young children with autism? Autism 2008;13(1):93-115.
[18] Yoder P, Stone WL. Randomized comparison of two communication interventions for preschoolers with autism spectrum disorders. J. Consult. Clin. Psychol. 2006;74(3):426-35.
[19] Luiselli JK, Cannon BOM, Ellis JT, Sisson RW. Home-based behavioral interventions for young children with autism/pervasive developmental disorder: A preliminary evaluation of outcome in relation to child age and intensity of service delivery. Autism 2000;4(4):426-38.
[20] Sheinkopf SJ, Siegel B. Home based behavioral treatment of young children with autism. J. Autism Dev. Disord 1998;28(1):15-23.
[21] Smith T, Buch GA, Gamby TE. Parent-directed, intensive early intervention for children with pervasive developmental disorder. Res. Dev. Disabil. 2000;21(4):297-309.
[22] Jordan R. Evaluating practice: Problems and possibilities. Autism 1999;3(4):411-34.
[23] Ruble L, Mathai G, Tanguay P, Josephson A, eds. Psychosocial treatment of Asperger's Disorder. NY: Informa Healthcare, 2008.
[24] Ruble, LA, Dalrymple NJ. An alternative view of outcome in autism. Focus Autism Other Dev. Disabil. 1996;11(1):3-14.
[25] Ruble LA, Dalrymple NJ. COMPASS: A parent-teacher collaborative model for students with autism. Focus Autism Other Dev. Disabil. 2002;17(2):76-83.
[26] Rue L, Dalrymple N, McGrew J. The effects of consultationon individualized education program outcomes for young children with autism: The collaborative model for promoting competence and success. J. of Early Intervnetion. 2010: 32(4):286-301.Ruble, L., Dalrymple, N., & McGrew. (2012). COMPASS: Providing Direction. Springer: NY.
[27] Mathai G, Ruble L. Implementing a social skills group for children with autism. J. Psychol. Pract. 2009;15:135-56.
[28] Nounopolous A, Ruble, L, Mathai G. Behavior management services for individuals with autism in an outpatient setting. J. Psychol. Pract. 2009;15:178-216.
[29] Mundy P, Burnette C. Joint attention and neurodevelopmental models of autism. Hoboken, NJ: John Wiley, 2005.
[30] Rajendran G, Mitchell P. Cognitive theories of autism. Dev. Rev 2007;27(2):224-60.
[31] Baron-Cohen S, Tager-Flusberg H, Cohen DJ. Understanding other minds. Perspectives from developmental cognitive neuroscience. 2nd ed. New York, NY: Oxford Univ Press, 2000.
[32] Frith U, Happe F. Autism: Beyond "theory of mind". Cognition 1994;50(1-3):115-32.
[33] Plaisted KC. Reduced generalization in autism. An alternative to weak central coherence. Mahwah, NJ: Lawrence Erlbaum, 2001.
[34] Denkla M. Biological correlates of learning and attention: What is relevant to learning disability and attention hyperactivity disorder? Dev. Behav. Paediatr. 1996;17:114-9.
[35] Lord C, McGee J. Educating children with autism. Washington, DC: Natl. Acad. Press, 2001.
[36] Smith T. Discrete trial training in the treatment of autism. Focus Autism Other Dev. Disabl. 2001;16(2):86-92.
[37] Rogers SJ. Play interventions for young children with autism spectrum disorders. Washington, DC: Am. Psychol. Assoc., 2005.
[38] Smith T, Mruzek DW, Peyton RT. A study in perseverance: The emergence of early intensive behavioral intervention. New York, NY: Springer, 2008.
[39] Lovaas OI, Smith T. Early and intensive behavioral intervention in autism. New York, NY: Guilford, 2003.
[40] Attwood T. Framework for behavioral interventions. Child Adolesc Psychiatr Clin. North Am. 2003;12(1):65-86.

[41] Fenske EC, Krantz PJ, McClannahan LE. Incidental teaching: A not-discrete-trial teaching procedure. Austin, TX: Pro-Ed, 2001
[42] Schreibman L, Koegel RL. Fostering self-management: Parent-delivered pivotal response training for children with autistic disorder. Washington, DC: Am. Psychol. Assoc., 1996.
[43] Schopler E, Mesibov GB, Hearsey K. Structured teaching in the TEACCH system. In: Schopler E, Mesibov GB. Learning and cognition in autism. Current issues in autism. New York, NY: Plenum, 1995:243-68.
[44] Jocelyn LJ, Casiro OG, Beattie D, Bow J, and Kneisz J. Treatment of children with autism: A randomized controlled trial to evaluate a caregiver-based intervention program in community day-care centers. Dev. Behav Pediatr. 1998;19:326-34.
[45] Drew A, Baird G, Baron-Cohen S, Cox A, Slonims V, Wheelwright S. A pilot randomized control trial of a parent training intervention for pre-school children with autism: Preliminary findings and methodological challenges. Eur. Child Adolesc. Psychiatr. 2002;11:266-72.
[46] Aldred C, Green J, Adams C. A new social communication intervention for children with autism: Pilot randomized controlled treatment study suggesting effectiveness. J. Child Psychol. Psychiatr. 2004;45:1420-30.
[47] Smith T, Groen AD, Wynn JW. Randomized trial of intensive early intervention for children with pervasive developmental disorder. Am. J. Ment. Retard. 2000;105:269-85.
[48] Sallows GO, Graupner TD. (2005) Intensive behavioral treatment for children with autism: Four-year outcome and predictors. Am. J. Ment. Retard. 2005;110:417-38.
[49] Bondy A, Frost L. The picture exchange communication system. Focus Autistic Behav. 1994;9(3):1-19.
[50] Happe F. Understanding assets and deficits in autism: Why success is more interesting than failure. Psychologist 1999;12:540-6.
[51] McClannahan L, Krantz P. Behavioral intervention for young children with autism: A manual for parents and professionals. Austin, TX: Pro-Ed, 1999.
[52] Stone W, Ruble L, Coonrod E, Hepburn S, Pennington M. TRIAD social skills assessment manual. Nashville, TN: Med Center South, 2002.
[53] Adams L, Gouvousis A, Vanlue M, Waldron C. Social story intervention: Improving communication skills in a child with Autism Spectrum Disorder. Focus Autism Other Dev Disabl 2003;19(2):87-94.
[54] Gray C, Garand J. Social Stories: Improving responses of students with autism with accurate social information. Focus Autistic Behav. 1993;8:1–10.
[55] Sansosti FJ, Powell Smith KA. Using social stories to improve the social behavior of children with Asperger syndrome. J. Positive Behav. Intervent. 2006;8(1):43-57.
[56] Baker, JE, Myles B. Social skills training for children and adolescents with Asperger syndrome and social-communication problems. Shawnee Mission, KS: Autism Asperger. Publ., 2003.
[57] Baker J. The social skills picture book: Teaching play, emotion and communication to children with autism. Arlington, TX: Future Horizons, 2001.
[58] Baker J. Social skills training for children and adolescents with Asperger Syndrome and social-communication problems. Shawnee Mission, KS: Autism Asperger Publ., 2003.
[59] Kendall PC. Child and adolescent therapy: Cognitive-behavioral procedures. 3rd ed. New York: Guilford, 2006.
[60] Schwartz, J. Brain Lock. New York: Harper Collins, 1996.
[61] McAfee J. Navigating the social world. Arlington, TX: Future Horizons, 2002.
[62] Kiresuk TJ, Smith A, Cardillo JE. Goal attainment scaling: Applications, theory, and measurement. Hillsdale, NJ: Lawrence Erlbaum, 1994.
[63] Marshall JK, Mirenda P. Parent–professional collaboration for positive behavior support in the home. Focus Autism other Dev. Disabl. 2002;17(4):216-28.
[64] Reinecke MA, Dattilio FM, Freeman A. Cognitive therapy with children and adolescents. A casebook for clinical practice. New York. Guilford, 2003.
[65] Buron KD, Curtis M. The Incredible 5-Point Scale. Shawnee Mission, KS: Autism Asperger Publ., 2003.

In: Understanding Autism Spectrum Disorder
Editors: Ditza A Zachor and Joav Merrick
ISBN: 978-1-62081-353-9

Chapter 6

Psychopharmacological treatment of ADHD symptoms in children with autism spectrum disorder

Benjamin L Handen, **Johanna Taylor and Rameshwari Tumuluru***
Western Psychiatric Institute and Clinic,
University of Pittsburgh School of Medicine,
Pittsburgh and Division of Special Education,
University of Pittsburgh,
Pennsylvania, United States

Abstract

One of the most frequently reported behavioral concerns among children with Autism Spectrum Disorder (ASD) is high rates of activity and inattention, symptoms that are often associated with Attention Deficit-Hyperactivity Disorder (ADHD). While there is a considerable body of research regarding the appropriate treatment of ADHD symptoms among typically developing children, the research among children with ASD is more limited.

The evidence to date suggests that medication response rates among children with ASD are considerably lower than among typically developing children and that children with ASD tend to be at greater risk for experiencing side effects. The purpose of the present chapter is to review the available research on the treatment of ADHD symptoms in children with ASD.

The chapter will summarize the data on a range of pharmacological options and provide specific recommendations for how best to clinically manage these symptoms.

* Correspondence: Benjamin L Handen, PhD, Western Psychiatric Institute and Clinic, 1011 Bingham St, Pittsburgh, PA 15203 United States. E-mail: handenbl@upmc.edu

Introduction

The pharmacological treatment of symptoms associated with Attention Deficit Hyperactivity Disorder (ADHD) has received considerable attention in the literature, dating back 3-4 decades. Recent large-scale controlled trials, such as the MTA, have confirmed the effectiveness of psychostimulants among typically developing children, with response rates of around 77%) (1) Other studies have demonstrated the efficacy of alternative medication classes to treat ADHD, including atomoxetine and alpha-two agonists. Children with Autism Spectrum Disorder (ASD), however, present a considerably more challenging picture for clinicians. ASD is characterized by significant deficits in communication skills, social interaction skills, and the presence of restricted repetitive behaviors or stereotypic interests (2). A recent survey of non-referred children with ASD found that symptoms suggestive of ADHD (e.g., distractibility, inattention, and fidgetiness) were reported in 60% of the sample by parents and in 40% of the sample by teachers (3). This same group of parents rated 41% of the children as moderately to severely hyperactive, while 29% were similarly rated by their teachers.

Surveys of medication prescribing rates in the United States have similarly found that treatment of ADHD symptoms to be among the most frequently identified target behavior. For example, Witwer and Lecavalier (4) examined psychotropic medication use in a non-referred sample of 353 school-age children with ASD and found that 24% had been prescribed stimulant medication in the past year.

Despite high rates of overactivity and inattention among children with ASD, DSM-IV2 specifically disallows a co-occurring diagnosis of ASD and ADHD: "The symptoms (of ADHD) do not occur exclusively during the course of a Pervasive Developmental Disorder" (p. 93). While two distinct disorders, ADHD and ASD have some areas of overlap. Symptoms common to both disorders include social skills deficits (e.g., poor peer relations, does not seem to listen when spoken to) as well as some similar neuropsychological deficits (e.g., problems with planning, working memory, inhibition, mental flexibility). In addition, both disorders are typically diagnosed at an early age and symptoms are often chronic, persisting into adulthood. Interestingly, many children diagnosed with Asperger's disorder or High Functioning Autism are often first diagnosed (or misdiagnosed) with ADHD.

Some ADHD theories posit dysregulation of norephinephrine and dopamine circuits, which results in deficits in areas of attention, executive function, and impulse control. However, it is unclear if the same deficits in children with ASD are due to similar neurotransmitter dysregulation. This may explain some differences in pharmacological treatment response rates.

The purpose of this paper is to provide an evidence-based strategy for the treatment of the child with ASD and symptoms of overactivity and inattention. This population presents a number of challenges to the treating clinician. First, overall response rates for children with ASD are considerably lower than among typically developing children. Second, even among responders, the level of improvement is often less robust. Third, side effects are more often reported, with significant numbers of children with ASD being unable to tolerate many of the medications commonly prescribed.

Interpretation of the research in this area can also be challenging. For example, there are often differences across studies regarding criteria used to diagnose both ADHD and ASD.

Studies utilize different definitions of "response" (e.g., ranging from 25% to 50% improvement over baseline).

Some studies only include children who meet diagnostic criteria for autistic disorder, while others include the entire autism spectrum. Finally, medication dose ranges are not necessarily consistent across studies. While this paper will focus on pharmacologic treatment options, psychosocial treatment should always be included as part of every child's overall treatment plan.

In addition, it is assumed that prior to initiating pharmacological treatment for ADHD symptoms that the clinician has conducted a reasonable assessment of the situation and determined that other factors, such as sleep problems, pain, family stress, etc. have been addressed.

This paper will review the literature on three primary medication classes that contain the best evidence of efficacy in this population, presenting them in the order of suggested consideration. Finally, we will discuss some other possible treatment options and the available supporting data.

First line treatment options

Stimulants

Stimulant medications are typically the first treatment option for individuals diagnosed with ADHD. They act on the norepinephrine and dopamine systems (by blocking reuptake at their respective transporters) and have led to the hypothesis that ADHD is a disorder related to catecholamine dysfunction (5).

Despite being the most studied class of medications among typically developing children, there have been few well-controlled studies of stimulants among children and adolescents with ASD. Only 10-15 years ago, the general sense among clinicians was that stimulants were often contraindicated for this population (6). This consensus was based upon a small number of case reports indicating a high rate of side effects and minimal treatment efficacy. Some of the earliest work with the ASD population was conducted by Campbell and her colleagues in which stimulant medications were found to increase stereotypic behavior and irritability in children with ASD (7,8). It should be noted that subjects were not specifically selected for hyperactivity. Since Campbell's work, there have been only slightly more than a dozen additional studies of stimulant use in children with ASD. The majority have involved case reports (9). Quintana et al (10) and Handen et al (11) conducted the only double-blind, placebo-controlled studies of methylphenidate (MPH) in children with ASD between 1990 and 2000. Both studies noted significant gains on measures of overactivity and inattention. Side effects, especially at higher doses, occurred more than in typically developing children and response rates were considerably lower than that found in the normal population. Stigler et al (12) published a retrospective study of 195 children and adolescents with ASD who had been prescribed stimulant medication at a hospital-based clinic. Only 24.6% of patients were considered to be responders to their first stimulant trial, with an even lower response rate among patients who were prescribed a second stimulant. Subjects with a diagnosis of Asperger's Disorder tended to have higher rates of response than children with Autism

Disorder or PDD Not Otherwise Specified. Additionally, high rates of adverse events were reported.

Finally, a relatively large, double-blind, placebo-controlled crossover study of MPH involving 72 children with ASD was recently published (13). The cross-over design included b.i.d. doses of 0.125, 0.25, and 0.5 mg and a smaller third dose in the afternoon. Forty-nine percent of subjects were responders, based upon a ≥30% decrease on either the parent or teacher-completed Hyperactivity subscale of the Aberrant Behavior Checklist (or a ≥25% decrease on both parent and teacher Hyperactivity subscales) and an improvement score of "1" or "2" on the Clinical Global Impressions Scale. However, 18% of subjects experienced adverse events so severe that they were forced to discontinue the study. Neither ASD diagnostic category nor IQ was found to be associated with treatment response.

The evidence suggests that MPH can be efficacious among some children with ASD and symptoms of ADHD, based upon the results of at least three double-blind, placebo controlled trials. However, response rates are lower than among typically developing children with ADHD and side effects are not uncommon (resulting in the need for discontinuation of medication of almost one fifth of children). There remain no recent studies of dextroamphetamine, mixed amphetamine salts (Adderall) or any of the current extended release stimulants in this population. However, there is no reason to assume that response rates should differ significantly from that reported with methylphenidate. Psychostimulants remain the first line of treatment for ADHD symptoms among children with ASD.

Atomoxetine

Atomoxetine (ATX) is a non-stimulant medication currently approved by the Food and Drug Administration (FDA) to treat individuals over the age of six with ADHD. This psychopharmacological option is considered an alternative drug to traditional stimulants (i.e., methylphenidate) and is typically prescribed one time per day. ATX's mechanism of action blocks the reuptake of norepinephrine, decreasing extreme activity levels and inattentiveness of individuals with ADHD (5). The use of ATX for typically developing children and adults is strongly supported by randomized controlled studies as an effective treatment for short and long-term use. It is well tolerated by subjects and produces minimal side effects (14). Response rates to ATX appear to be similar to immediate release MPH but somewhat less effective than osmotically-released MPH or extended release mixed amphetamine salts. (14) Despite evidence of efficacy of ATX among typically developing children with ADHD, there have been relatively few studies of this agent's use among children with ASD.

We are aware of three open-label studies reporting the use of ATX to treat ADHD symptoms in children with ASD. Jou et al (15) conducted a retrospective chart review of 20 individuals with ASD (ages 6-19 years), half of whom also had intellectual disability. The majority were also prescribed concomitant medications to address behavioral concerns. Doses ranged from 25 mg to 80 mg (mean 43.3 mg) and the length of the trial ranged from 1 to 36 weeks (mean 19.5 weeks). Twelve of the 20 subjects experienced significant decreases in symptoms of hyperactivity and inattentiveness on the CPRS from baseline to completion (17.1 to 13.0 and 7.5 to 5.8, respectively). Mild to moderate side effects were reported, with one subject discontinuing medication due to severe mood swings. Troost et al (16) conducted a prospective, open-label study of 12 children (ages 6-14 years) with ASD (6 autistic disorder,

5 PDD-not otherwise specified, and 1 Asperger's disorder). All subjects had borderline to normal intellectual functioning. Subjects discontinued all concomitant medications prior to the trial. A flexible dosing schedule was used for this 10-week trial. Final doses ranged from 17.5 to 80mg. Statistically significant decreases were noted on the Hyperactivity subscale and ADHD Index of the Conners' Parent Rating Scale-Revised as well as Clinical Global Impressions (CGI) ratings of ADHD severity. However, five children were removed from the study prematurely due to an increase in gastrointestinal problems.

A third study was conducted by Posey et al (17) and prospectively assessed the effectiveness of ATX in 17 children and adolescents (ages 6-17) with ASD. All subjects were free of any commitment psychotropic medications at the time of study entry. Thirteen subjects completed the treatment protocol (two were discontinued due to inability to swallow pills and two due to irritability). Mean dose was 1.2 mg per day. Parent and teacher reports indicated statistically significant decreases on the SNAP-IV Hyperactivity-Impulsivity subscale and the Hyperactivity subscale of the Aberrant Behavior Checklist (18)(ABC)(28.4 ± 8.5 to 14.2 ± 6.6). However, no statistically significant change was noted on the Conners' Continue Performance Test (19). One subject experienced both gastrointestinal problems and blunted affect.

The only existing double-blind, placebo-controlled study of ATX was a conducted by Arnold et al (20) with a group of 16 children with ASD (ages 5-15 years). Subjects were allowed to continue concomitant medications (except ß-blockers and systemic drugs), providing doses were constant one month prior to baseline. A cross-over design was used with doses ranging from 20 mg to 100 mg (mean highest dose = 44.2 ± 21.9 mg/day). Each condition was conducted for six weeks, with dose titration during the first three weeks. The parent ABC and a rating scale of DSM-IV ADHD symptoms indicated a statistically significant difference from baseline after six weeks of treatment (ABC Hyperactivity: 24.69 to 19.31; DSM-IV Hyperactivity: 17.31 to 10.40). Similar to the Troost et al (16) study, a high rate of gastrointestinal problems were reported. In addition, 12 subjects reported fatigue and one child was discontinued four weeks into the active medication arm of the trial due to a severe adverse event.

Alpha-2-adrenergic receptor agonists

Alpha-2-adrenergic agonists reduce arousal by inhibiting the locus coeruleus. This appears to decrease norepinephrine function, which in turn, reduces hyperactivity. The dopaminergic and serotonerigc systems are also affected, which may improve attention (21,22). The alpha-2-adrenergic agonists, clonidine (Catapres) and guanfacine (Tenex), have been used alone and in combination with stimulants for a number of years to decrease symptoms of ADHD. However, neither agent has been FDA approved for such purpose (having been approved as anti-hypertensives). The former has also been shown to be efficacious for the treatment of Tourette's syndrome in controlled, multicenter trials (23). There have also been a few small trials of clonidine and guanfacine for the treatment of ADHD symptoms in ASD. For example, Jaselskis et al (24) conducted a double-blind, placebo-controlled, crossover trial of clonidine in a group of eight children diagnosed with ASD (ages 2.8 to 8.1 years). Doses were gradually increased to 0.15-0.20 mg/day (three dosages per day) during the first two weeks of treatment and held steady for the subsequent four weeks. During weeks 6 and 7, the medication was tapered. Subjects were then titrated in a manner similar to weeks 1-6 (with either placebo or active medication). Teacher ratings resulted in statistically significant (but not clinically significant) improvement on the Hyperactivity subscale of the ABC (placebo, 28.4 ± 10.8; clonidine 24.9 ± 11.1). Similar findings occurred using the Connors Parent-Teacher Questionnaire (placebo = 12.9 ± 5.5; clonidine = 10.1 ± 4.9). Clonidine doses were decreased in three subjects due to side effects (e.g., hypotension, drowsiness). Fankhauser et al (25) used a clonidine transdermal patch in a double-blind, crossover study of nine individuals with ASD (ages 5-33 years). Significant improvement on measures of socially relating to people, affectual responses, and sensory responses were noted, as well as modest improvement on the CGI scale for overactivity.

Posey et al (26) retrospectively examined the effects of guanfacine in a chart review of 80 individuals (ages 3 to 18 years) with ASD (28 PDD-NOS; six Asperger's disorder; 46 Autistic Disorder). The average duration of treatment was 334 days (range 7-1,776 days). Only 23.8% of subjects were determined to be responders, based upon improvement of symptoms such as hyperactivity, inattention, insomnia, and tics. The most frequently reported side effect was transient sedation (31.3%). Other side effects such as irritability, nocturnal enuresis, headache, and constipation were reported by 15.1% of subjects.

Scahill et al (27) conducted an eight-week open-label prospective study of guanfacine in a sample of 25 children with ASD (mean age = 3.14 ± 9.0). All subjects had been nonresponsive to a prior trial of methylphenidate. Medication was titrated over a 5-week period to a maximum of 3.0 mg/day (in 2 or 3 divided doses).

Parents reported a 39% decrease on the Hyperactivity subscale of the ABC and a 36% decrease on the SNAP-IV. Slightly less improvement was seen on the teacher ABC Hyperactivity subscale (27% decrease) and teacher SNAP-IV (18%). The most common side effects requiring dose adjustment or reduction were sedation, irritability and sleep disturbance. Three subjects discontinued the trial due to irritability.

The only existing double blind, placebo-controlled study for children with ASD and symptoms of ADHD was conducted by Handen, Sahl and Harden (28). Eleven children (ages 5 to 9 years) were diagnosed with intellectual disability and/or ASD and seven were taking other stabilized medications during the treatment phase. Eight participants accepted the maximum dose of 3 mg/day. The other three subjects received lower doses (1.0 to 2.5 mg/day) due to AEs.

Five subjects were named "medication responders," which was indicated by a decrease of ≥50% on the parent and teacher ABC hyperactivity subscale. Hyperactivity was the only symptom that decreased. Three of the children (27%) had AEs and dose titration ceased prior to the completion of the study. The most commonly reported side effects were fatigue and lethargic behavior with diarrhea, social withdrawal, and constipation also observed.

Recently, guanfacine-extended release formulation (GXR: Intuniv) was FDA approved for the treatment of ADHD in children and adolescents ages 6-17 years as a monotherapy (however, short acting guanfacine remains "off-label" when used to treat ADHD).

Two large, multicenter controlled trials have been published documenting this agent's efficacy among typically developing children with ADHD. The first was an 8-week trial conducted by Biederman et al (29) involving 345 children (ages 6 to17) with age appropriate intellectual ability and ADHD. The second study by Sallee et al (30) investigated the use of GXR with 324 children (ages 6 to 17) over a nine week period. Both studies reported significant improvements on the ADHD-RS-IV rating scale. Side effects included sedation, dizziness, and fatigue. There is no published data regarding the use of GXR among children with ASD.

Other medications options

For children with ASD who fail to respond to stimulants, atomoxetine, or alpha-two adrenergic agonists, the options are somewhat limited. One possibility are the use of the atypical antipsychotic, risperidone or aripiprazole. Risperidone and aripiprazole are the only pharmacological agent currently approved for the US Food and Drug Administration for treatment of irritability in ASD. While not recommended as a treatment for ADHD behaviors in ASD per se, if risperidone or aripiprazole are being considered for use due to concerns with a child's aggression or irritability, there is some evidence that ADHD symptoms will be similarly affected. In a 2002 New England Journal of Medicine paper, the Research Units on Pediatric Psychopharmacology in Autism reported the results of a multi-center, placebo-controlled, double-blind trial of risperidone for irritability in ASD (31). A 69% response rate was found, based upon a 25% decrease on the Irritability subscale of the ABC and an improvement score of "1" or "2" on the CGI Severity Rating Scale. The Hyperactivity subscale of the ABC also evidenced similar gains, with a mean decrease of 46.5% for the active medication group versus 14.5% for placebo. A second, placebo-controlled Canadian trial of risperidone in ASD found similar results, with a mean decrease of 54.6% on the ABC Hyperactivity subscale for the risperidone group in comparison to 23.9% for those on placebo (32). A controlled trial of aripiprazole in ASD was recently completed. Results indicated significant improvement on measures of irritability in comparison to placebo. In addition, significant decreases were noted on the Hyperactivity subscale of the ABC (using fixed doses of 5, 10 and 15 mg/day) in comparison to placebo (33).

There has been increasing interest in agents that affect the glutamatergic system, as there is some evidence that abnormalities of the glutamate receptors and transporters in the cerebellum may be involved in pathophysiology of ASD (34) King et al (35) first reported the results of an open-label study of amantadine in a group eight children with neuro-developmental disorders (two of who had ASD). Amantadine is an N-methyl-D-aspartate (NMDA) receptor antagonist and indirect dopamine agonist. Doses ranged from 3.7 to 8.2 mg/kg/day. Outcomes were limited to subjective clinical ratings and found four subjects to be responders, based upon decreasing on symptoms such as hyperactivity, impulsivity and aggression. However, a subsequent, multi-center, placebo-controlled, double-blind study involving 39 children and adolescents with ASD failed to support the findings of the open-label trail. There has also been a long-standing interest in the use of naltrexone, an opiate antagonist, for the treatment of self-injurious behavior in ASD. It was hypothesized that higher levels of beta-endorphins found among individuals with ASD may be related to dysfunctional modulation of proopiomelanocortin peptides and serotonin by the pineal-hypothalamic-pituitary-adrenal axis (37). However, the research in support of naltrexone as an effective treatment for self-injurious behavior has been equivocal (37)). Other studies have examined naltrexone's affect on symptoms of ADHD. However, Kolmen et al (38,39) conducted two controlled trials in a total of 24 young children with ASD and found only modest gains on measures of attention and overactivity. Consequently, neither amantadine nor naltrexone is typically considered as strong alternative options for treating ADHD symptoms in the ASD population.

The research on the use of antimanics among children with ASD has been fairly limited, with most trials targeting behaviors such as disruption or aggression. We are aware of only three published controlled trials involving individuals with ASD. Of these, a study of lamotrigine failed to show any difference between placebo and active medication on measures of hyperactivity and attention (40) and a study of valproate failed to find any difference between placebo and active medication on measures of irritability (no measures of hyperactivity or inattention were reported) (41). Only a controlled trial of divalproex sodium found significant decreases on measures of repetitive behaviors. However, no measures of inattention or overactivity were used. At present, there does not appear to be enough data to support the use of antimanics to treat ADHD symptoms in this population.

Finally, there has been some recent interest in cholinesterase inhibitors as possible treatment for both core and secondary features of ASD. The interest in this class of agents is based upon findings of pathological abnormalities in the basal forebrain (septal) cholinergic neurons among individuals with ASD (42). Neurochemical abnormalities in the cholinergic system have also been documented in ASD, including decreases in cortical M1 receptors in the parietal cortex, nicotinic receptors in the parietal and frontal cortices, and alpha4 and beta2 nicotinic receptor subunits in the parietal cortex (43). A retrospective study of 8 children (ages 7-19 years) with autism who had been prescribed donepezil (mean dose 9.37 mg/day) was conducted by Hardan and Handen (44). Half of the subjects were deemed responders, based upon statistically significant reductions on the Irritability and Hyperactivity subscales of the Aberrant Behavior Checklist.

Mild, transient side effects were reported, including vomiting and increased irritability. Chez et al (45) conducted a controlled trial of donepezil (2.5 mg/day) in 43 children (ages 2-10 years) with ASD. He reported significant gains in receptive and expressive language skills as well as improvement on measures of the core features of autism (CARS: Childhood Autism Rating Scale). However, no measures of ADHD symptoms were utilized. Interpretation of the results were further complicated as no between group statistical analyses were conducted and on some measures the placebo group displayed greater improvement than the active medication group (46).

Handen et al (47) recently reported the results of a double-blind, placebo-controlled trial of donepezil in a group of 34 children and adolescents with ASD (does of 5 mg and 10 mg/day). While the placebo group evidenced a greater decrease on the Inattention and ADHD subscales of the Child Behavior Checklist than subjects on active medication, no statistically significant between group differences were found. Finally, Chez et al (48) reported the results of an open label trial of rivastigmine in a group of 32 children with ASD (0.8 mg twice daily).

Improvement was noted on the Connors scale (i.e., ADHD symptoms), measures of expressive language, and on core features of autism. Memantine, another cognitive enhancing agent that has been approved for treatment of Alzheimer's disease, has also experienced recent interest as a possible treatment in ASD.

A moderate antagonist, memantine binds to NMDA receptors and blocks glutamate access to cells (49). Chez (50) recently report findings of the use of memamtine as an add-on therapy for 151 patients with ASD (age range 2.58 to 25.33 years). Doses ranged from 2.5 to t0 30 mg/day (mean 12.67 mg). Statistically significant gains were reported using Clinical Global Impressions scores for language, self-stimulatory behavior, and general behavior. However, the CGI-I for behavior was focused on gains in social interactions, cooperation, and following directions. Consequently, it is not known what affect memantine may have had on overactivity and inattention. With the exception of atypical antipsychotics (especially risperidone), the evidence supporting the efficacy of alternative agents to treat ADHD symptoms in ASD is fairly weak.

Conclusion

In summary, there is considerable support for the treatment of ADHD in the typically developing population. However, the extant literature is more limited in children with ASD. This limitation may be explained by various factors, including the exclusion of children with ASD in most large studies, the exclusion of ADHD as a co-morbid disorder for children with ASD (per DSM-IV guidelines), and earlier reports that the use of stimulants with this population was contraindicated. Despite this, there has been more interest in the treatment of overactivity and inattention in individuals with ASD. However, the rate and robustness of treatment response may be less than that seen among typically developing children. Side effects are also more likely to occur, and concerns remain regarding cardiotoxicity with the use of stimulants and ATX, as well as increased suicidal ideation with ATX for both the typical and ASD population (51,52). The first line treatment should be with the use of stimulant medication, where at least three of double-blind, placebo-controlled trials have been conducted. The support for alternative options, such as ATX, is limited to a handful of open-label studies and a single double-blind, placebo-controlled trial. The use of alpha-two agonists also has some research support in ASD, with a group of small, double-blind trials having been conducted. Once the use of stimulants, ATX and alpha-two agonists are found not be efficacious for an individual with ASD, there is strong support for the use of risperidone or aripiprazole. These two agents have been evaluated in a number of large, multi-center controlled trials for the treatment of irritability in ASD. However, secondary effects on measures of hyperactivity were also robust. This option should be reserved, however, for individuals who also present with either symptoms of irritability or severe overactivity and impulsivity that has not responded to other pharmacologic treatment. Finally, there is limited support at this time for the use of antimanics, naltrexone or amantadine for the treatment of ADHD. Some increasing interest in the use of cognitive enhancing agents, such as cholinesterase inhibitors, may lead to additional data on the effects of this class of drugs on activity and attention.

References

[1] Greenhill LL, Swanson JM, Vitiello B, Davies M, Clevenger W, Wu M, et al. Impairment and deportment responses to different methylphenidate doses in children with ADHD: the MTA titration trial. J. Am. Acad. Child Adolesc. Psychiatry 2007;40:180-7.

[2] American Psychiatric Association, Diagnostic and statistical manual of mental disorders, 5th ed. Washington, DC: APA, 2000.

[3] Lecavalier, L. Behavior and emotional problems in young people with pervasive developmental disorders: Relevant prevalence, effects of subject characteristics, and empirical classification. J. Autism Dev. Disord. 2006;36:1101-14.

[4] Witwer A, Levavalier L. Treatment incidence and patterns in children and adolescents with autism spectrum disorders. J. Child Adolesc. Psychopharmacology 2005;15:671-81.

[5] Pliszka SR. The nejuropsychopharmacology of attention-deficit/hyperactivity disorder. Biol. Psychiatry 2005;57:1385-90.

[6] Aman, MG. Stimulant drugs in the developmental disabilities revisited. J. Dev. Phys. Disabil. 1996;4:347-66.

[7] Campbell M. Pharmacotherapy in early infantile autism. Biol. Psychiatry 1975;10:399-423.

[8] Campbell M, Cohen I. Treatment of infantile autism. Compr. Ther. 1978;4:33-7.

[9] Di Martino A, Melis G, Cianchetti C, Zuddas A. Methylphenidate for pervasive developmental disorders: Safety and efficacy of acute single dose test and ongoing therapy: An open-pilot study. J Child Adolesc Psychopharmacology 2004;14:207-18.

[10] Quintana H, Birmaher B, Stedge D, Lennon S, Freed J, Bridge J. Use of methylphenidate in the treatment of children with autistic disorder. J. Autism Dev. Disorder. 1995;25: 283-94.

[11] Handen BL, Johnson CR, Lubetsky M. Efficacy of methylphenidate among children with autism and symptoms of attention-deficit hyperactivity disorder. J. Autism Dev. Disord. 2000;30:245-55.

[12] Stigler KA, Desmond LA, Posey DJ et al : A naturalistic retrospective analysis of psychostimulants in pervasive developmental disorders. J. Child adolesc. Psychopharmacol. 2004;14:49-56.

[13] RUPP. Randomized, controlled, crossover trial of methylphenidate in pervasive developmental disorders with hyperactivity. Arch. Gen. Psychiatry 2005;62:1266-74.

[14] Garnock-Jones, Karly P. Keating, Gillian M. Atomoxetine: a review of its use in attention-deficit hyperactivity disorder in children and adolescents. Paediatric Drugs 2009;11:203-26.

[15] Jou RJ, Handen BL, Hardan AY. Retrospective assessment of atomoxetine in children and adolescents with pervasive developmental disorders. J. Child Adolesc. Psychopharmacology 2005;15:325-30.

[16] Troost PW, Althaus M, Lahuis BE, Buitelaar JK, Minderaa RB, Hoekstra PJ. Neuropsychological effects of risperidone in children with pervasive developmental disorders: A blinded discontinuation study. J. Child Adolesc. Psychopharmacology 2006;16:561-73.

[17] Posey DJ, Wiegand RE, Wilkerson J, Maynard M, Stigler KA, McDougles CJ. Open-label atomoxetine for attention-deficit/hyperactivity disorder symptoms associated with high-functioning pervasive developmental disorders. J. Child Adolesc. Psychopharmacology 2006;16:599-610.

[18] Aman MG, Singh NN, Stewart AW, Field, CJ (1985). The Aberrant Behavior Checklist: A behavior rating scale for the assessment of treatment effects. American Journal of Mental Deficiency, 89, 485-491.

[19] Conners CK: Conners' Continuous Performance Test—II. North Tonawanda, NY: Multi-Health Systems, 2000.

[20] Arnold LE, Aman MG, Cook A, Witwer A, Hall K, Thompson S, Ramadan Y. Atomoxetine for hyperactivity in autistic spectrum disorders: Placebo-controlled crossover trial. J. Am. Acad. Child Adolesc. Psychiatry 2006;45:1196-1205.

[21] Werry JS, Aman MG. Practitioner's guide to psychoactive drugs for children and adolescents, 2nd ed. New York: Plenum Med Book, 1999.

[22] Poncin Y, Scahill L. Stimulants and nonstimulants in the treatment of hyperactivity in autism. In: Hollander E, Anagnostou E, eds., Clinical manual for the treatment of autism. Washington DC: Am. Psychiatr. Publ., 2007:131-52.

[23] Tourette's Syndrome Study Group: Treatment of ADHD in children with tics: A randomized controlled trial. Neurology 2002;58:527-36.

[24] Jaselskis CA, Cook EH, Fletcher KE, Leventhal B. Clonidine treatment of hyperactivity and impulsive children with autistic disorder. J. Clin. Psychopharmacology 1992;12:322-6.

[25] Fankhasuer MP, Karumanchi VC, German ML et al : A double-blind, placebo-controlled study of the efficacy of transdermal clonidine in autism. J. Clin. Psychiatry 1992;53:77-82.

[26] Posey DJ, Puntney JI, Sasher TM, Kem DL, McDougle CJ. Guanfacine treatment of hyperactivity and inattention in pervasive developmental disorders: A retrospective analysis of 80 cases. J. Child Adolesc. Psychopharmacology 2004;14:233-41.

[27] Scahill L, Aman MG, McDougle CJ, McCracken JT, Tierney E, Dziura J, et al. A prospective open trial of guanfacine in children with pervasive developmental disorders. J. Child Adolesc. Psychopharmacology 2006;16:589-598.

[28] Handen BL, Sahl R, Harden AY. Guanfacine in children with autism and/or intellectual disabilities. J. Dev. Behav. Pediatr. 2008;29:303-8.

[29] Biederman J. Melmed RD. Patel A. McBurnett K. Konow J. Lyne A. Scherer N. A randomized, double-blind, placebo-controlled study of guanfacine extended release in children and adolescents with attention-deficit/hyperactivity disorder. Pediatrics. 2008;121(1):e73-84.

[30] Sallee FR. Lyne A. Wigal T. McGough JJ. Long-term safety and efficacy of guanfacine extended release in children and adolescents with attention-deficit/hyperactivity disorder. J. Child Adolesc. Psychopharmacology 2009;19:215-26.

[31] McCracken JT, McGough J, Shah B, Cronin P, Hong D, Aman MG, et al. Research Units on Pediatric Psychopharmacology Autism Network. Risperidone in children with autism and serious behavioral problems. New Engl. J. Med. 2002;347:314-21.

[32] Shea S, Turgay A, Carrol A, Schulz M, Orlik H, Smith I. Risperidone in the treatment of disruptive behavioral symptoms in children with autistic and other pervasive developmental disorders. Am. J. Psychiatry 2004;161:2115-7.

[33] Marcus RN, Owen R, Kamen L, Manos, G, McQuade RD, Carson W, Aman MG. A placebo-controlled, fixed-dose study of aripiprazole in children and adolescents with irritability associated with autistic disorder. J. Am. Acad. Child Adolesc. Psychiatry 2009;48:1110-9.

[34] Purcell AE, Jeon OH, Zimmerman AW, Blue ME, Pevsner J. Postmortem brain abnormalities of the glutamate neurotransmitter system in autism. Neurology 2001;57(9):1618-28.

[35] King BH, Wright, M, Snape M, Dourish CT. Case Series: Amantadine open-label treatment of impulsive and aggressive behavior in hospitalized children with developmental disabilities. J. Am. Acad. Child Adolesc. Psychiatry 2001;40:654-7.

[36] King BH, Wright DM, Handen BL, et al. A double-blind, placebo-controlled study of amantadine hydrochloride in the treatment of children with autistic disorder. J. Am. Acad. Child Adolesc. Psychiatry 2001,;40:658-65.

[37] Chamberlain RS, Herman BH. A novel biochemical model linking dysfunctions in brain melatonin, proopiomelanocortin peptides, and serotonin in autism. Biol. Psychiatry 1990;28:773-93.

[38] Kolmen BK, Feldman H, Handen BL, Janosky JE. Naltrexone in young autistic children: A double blind placebo-controlled crossover study. J. Am. Academy Child Adolesc. Psychiatry 1995;34:223-31.

[39] Kolmen BK, Feldman HM, Handen BL, Janosky JE. Naltrexone in young autistic children: Replication study and learning measures. J. Am. Acad. Child Adolesc. Psychiatry 1997;36:1570-8.

[40] Belsito KM, Law PA, Kirk KS, Landa RJ, Zimmerman AW. Lamotrigine therapy for autistic disorder: a randomized, double-blind, placebo-controlled trial. J. Autism Dev. Disord. 2001;31:175-81.

[41] Hellings JA, Weckbaugh M, Nickel EJ, Cain S, Zarcone J, Reese RM, et al. A double-blind, placebo-controlled study of valproate for aggression in youth with pervasive developmental disorders. J. Child Adolesc. Psychopharmacology 2005;15:682-92.

[42] Bauman ML, Kemper TL. Neuroanatomic observations of the brain in autism. In: Bauman M , Kemper T. The neurobiology of autism. Baltimore, MD: Johns Hopkins Univ Press, 1994:119-145.

[43] Perry E, Lee M, Martin-Ruiz C, Court J, Volsen S, Merrit J, et al. Cholinergic activity in autism: Abnormalities in the cerebral cortex and basal forebrain. Am. J. Psychiatry 2001;158:1058-66.

[44] Hardan AY, Handen BL. A retrospective open trial of adjunctive donepezil in children and adolescents with autistic disorder. J. Child Adolesc. Psychopharmacology 2002;12:237-42.

[45] Chez MG, Buchanan TM, Becker M, Kessler J, Aimonovitch MC, Mrazek SR. Donepezil hydrochloride: A double-blind study in autistic children. J. Pediatric Neurology 2003;1:83–8.

[46] Yoo HJ, Valdovinos HG, Williams DC. Relevance of donepezil in enhancing learning and memory in special populations: A Review of the Literature. J. Autism Dev. Disord. 2007;37:1883-1901.
[47] Handen BL, Johnson CR, McAuliffe-Bellin S, Hardan AO. Safety and efficacy of donepezil in children and adolescents with autism: Behavioral measures. Int. Public Health J., in press.
[48] Chez MG, Aimonovitch M, Buchanan T, Mrazek S, Tremb RJ. Treating autistic spectrum disorders in children: utility of the cholinesterase inhibitor rivastigmine tartrate. J. Child Neurology 2004;19:165-9.
[49] Parsons CG, Danysz W, Quack G. Memantine is a clinically well tolerated N-methyl-D-aspartate (NMDA) receptor antagonist: a review of preclinical data. Neuropharmacology 1999;38:735-67.
[50] Chez MG. Burton Q. Dowling T. Chang M. Khanna P. Kramer C. Memantine as adjunctive therapy in children diagnosed with autistic spectrum disorders: an observation of initial clinical response and maintenance tolerability. J. Child Neurology 2007;22:574-9.
[51] Bangs ME, Tauscher-Wisniewsk S, Polzer J, Zhang, S, Acharya N, Deshaiah D, et al. Meta-analysis of suicide-related behavior events in patients treated with atomoxetine. J. Am. Acad. Child Adolesc. Psychiatry 2008;47:209-18.
[52] McCarthy S, Cranswick N, Potts, L, Taylor E, Wong IC. Mortality associated with attention-deficit hyperactivity disorder (ADHD) drug treatment: A retrospective cohort study of children, adolescents and young adults using the General Practice Research Database. Drug. Sat. 2009;32:1089-96.

In: Understanding Autism Spectrum Disorder
Editors: Ditza A Zachor and Joav Merrick

ISBN: 978-1-62081-353-9

Chapter 7

Enhancing multidisciplinary community supports for minority preschool children with autistic spectrum disorders: Promoting family centered and evidence based practices

Valeria Nanclares-Nogues[1], Elaine Lin[2], Carol Rolland[1], J. Michael Cupoli[1] and Michael E. Msall[2]

[1]Pediatric Developmental Center,
Advocate Illinois Masonic Medical Center,
Chicago, Illinois
[2]Section of Developmental and Behavioral Pediatrics,
Kennedy Research Center on Intellectual
and Developmental Disabilities,
University of Chicago Comer and La Rabida Children's Hospitals,
Chicago, Illinois, United States

Abstract

Our objective was to compare functional profiles of preschool children with autism to other preschool developmental delays and measure parental priorities. We piloted a comprehensive treatment program to address these priorities in resource-scarce settings. In Phase 1,230 children ages 1-3 years completed standardized assessments of communicative, social-emotional, and adaptive skills. Structured interviews for family priorities were completed. In Phase 2, a 25-hour community-based treatment program (PUENTES) for preschool children with autism was undertaken to enhance communicative, behavioral, and adaptive skills. Assessments at baseline included the Psychoeducational Profile-R (PEP-R), Vineland Adaptive Behavior Scales (VABS), and Parental Sense of Competence Scale (PSCS). Assessments were repeated after 4 months.

Of the 230 children, 199 were diagnosed with autism, 83 with mixed developmental disorder, and 48 with global developmental delay. Children with autism had the most difficulties in communication and adaptive behavior. Across all groups, parents' initial priorities were getting services (77%) and understanding children's needs (71%). Of the families seen in follow-up, 60% experienced high levels of stress, and 33% reported high rates of difficulty obtaining supports. Only 50% of parents rated their own physical health as excellent/very good. Among the 20 children in PUENTES, major gains in all developmental skills occurred. All pre and post changes on PEPS-R, VABS, and PSCS were significant. Parents reported that their participation facilitated their children's learning and enhanced their sense of competency. Our pilot data indicate that a collaborative program that bridges home, school, and community services is effective for preschool children with autism.

Introduction

Autism spectrum disorder (ASD) is an early onset neurodevelopmental disorder characterized by impairments in communication, social functioning, and adaptive behaviors. There is a general consensus that increasing numbers of young children are being diagnosed with autistic spectrum disorder with current overall prevalence rate at 60-70 per 10,000 (1-5).

In the past decade, major policy statements by the American Academy of Pediatrics and the National Academy of Sciences have provided a template for widely disseminated state of the art strategies for diagnosis and management (6-8). However, there are substantial gaps between these guidelines and families' goals of feeling supported and their children accessing quality and comprehensive early education services (9-11). In addition, developing effective and accessible services for children with autism is difficult because the disorder itself is complex, heterogeneous, and requires intensive intervention across multiple developmental dimensions and settings (12-16).

In developing guidelines from available scientific studies and expert opinions, Lord and McGee concluded that at least 25 hours per week of systematically planned and developmentally appropriate activity toward identified treatment objectives is required to effectively intervene with autism (6).

These levels of service are often not available to families, particularly for young children with autism living in resource-limited urban communities. While the public schools in most states are mandated to provide educational intervention for children with autism for children in the 3-6 year age range, total service hours often do not reach the 25-hour level. In addition, procedures for assuring treatment integrity may not be present in traditional special educational settings, particularly in terms of delivery of appropriate hours of systematic, data-based, objective interventions with the child.

Families often choose to enlist private therapists to work with their children, at times contracting for as many as 30-40 hours of weekly home-based therapy.

While child outcome data for these intensive behavioral approaches have shown significant gains, these therapies can be prohibitively expensive, and may cost over $50,000 per year (17,18).

Costs at this level are out of the reach of most families, and it remains unclear whether these intensive behavioral treatments (IBT) represent the most effective approach for children – i.e., if there may be other effective treatment options for families (19-21).

A number of treatment approaches have reported significant changes in selected outcome measures for children and adolescents with autism. Several have focused on behavioral skills, such as the intensive behavioral treatment (IBT) approaches (22-24), special educational practices such as the Treatment and Education of Autistic and related Communication-handicapped Children (TEACCH) model (25), language and communication-based interventions such as The Picture Exchange Communication System (PECS) (26), or Social Communication Emotional Regulation Transactional Support (SCERTS) (27).

Practitioners have proposed that programming which integrates various approaches shows the greatest likelihood for overall positive outcomes; however, there is little data to support this assertion (28-30).

The first phase of our study consisted of examining how adaptive skills impact parental stress and parental priorities in young urban preschoolers with autism. Adaptive behavior has been defined as one's ability to perform tasks of daily living and fulfill social roles expected of peers of the same age and culture, and several studies have documented how children with autism face challenges in this domain (31-32). Research among older children with global developmental delay and developmental language disorders has demonstrated how difficulties in communication interfere with the acquisition of adaptive skills (33). Because some of the hallmarks of autism are obstacles in learning social, adaptive, and communicative skills, functional assessment in preschool children with autism was assessed to determine appropriate interventions and supports that will address parents' concerns about daily management.

Our second phase of the study was designed to determine if a collaborative parent-therapist, integrated treatment approach for young children with autism could optimize learning, adaptive skills, and parental sense of competency. The treatment program was developed at an urban Chicago medical center to address families' needs for effective, affordable treatment for their young children with autism in a setting of limited resources (34). To maintain intensity levels while reducing overall costs, parents were trained to actively collaborate with the therapists, providing a substantial portion of the intervention (10 hours per week). The professional therapists provided on-going training and guidance for families as well as some of the direct therapy for the children (five hours per week). The preschool educational programs and habilitative therapies (OT, ST) provided an additional 10 hours of service.

To enhance clinical efficacy, we integrated a number of approaches that have demonstrated evidence of effectiveness for children with autism, including IBT and special educational approaches. This more "integrative" model allowed us to take advantage of the strengths of each approach and to individualize our treatment based on the children's unique learning styles. Although a number of studies combining treatment approaches have utilized the term "eclectic", we have preferred to use the term "integrative" in this paper, as we feel that our model has carefully and thoughtfully integrated the various approaches into a comprehensive treatment modality and is not simply a loose combination of approaches.

We hypothesized that this integrative intervention would increase children's developmental skills in communication, social, adaptive, and learning domains, as well as increase parental sense of competency.

First study

Parental stress, priorities and adaptive skills in young children with autistic spectrum disorder (ASD)

A retrospective chart review was conducted for 230 patients ages 0-5 years who were seen in the diagnostic clinics by the Developmental and Behavioral Section of Pediatrics at the University of Chicago between 2001 and 2005. All patients were referred by a pediatrician or Early Intervention service coordinator. Patients received a comprehensive evaluation that included administration of standardized developmental tests to assess gross and fine motor skills, receptive and expressive language skills, adaptive skills, and cognitive and problem solving skills. All parents initially completed surveys regarding parent stress and family priorities. Participants were included if data were available that described the child's health, development, and functioning regardless of developmental diagnosis. Children were excluded if data was not available to establish developmental functioning in communication or adaptive skills and a clinical review removed any children with incomplete or erroneous data.

The diagnosis of autism was given based on Diagnostic and Statistical Manual of Mental Disorders (DSM-IV) criteria and included the Modified Checklist for Autism in Toddlers, Childhood Autism Rating Scales, Autism Diagnostic Observation Scale, and the Gilliam Asperger Disorder Scales. Children diagnosed with Asperger's syndrome and pervasive developmental disorder-not otherwise specified were also included in this category. Children were classified as global developmental delay if they performed at a standard score (SS) of 70 or less in verbal, problem solving, and adaptive skills. Children were classified as a mixed developmental disorder if they had some score above 70 but multiple delays in motor, communicative, problem solving, or adaptive skills. All families consented to participate in multidisciplinary diagnosis and follow-up.

Measures

In Phase 1, communicative skills were assessed using the Receptive Expressive Emergent Language Scale-2, the Rossetti Infant Toddler Language Scale, or the Clinical Linguistic and Auditory Milestone Scale. Adaptive skills were measured using the Vineland Adaptive Behavior Scales Survey form. The Vineland outcome domains chosen for this study were Communication, Socialization, and Daily Living skills. If Vineland interviews were not available, the adaptive skills of the Battelle Developmental Inventory or the Self –Care Domain score of the Pediatric Functional Independence Measure (Wee-FIM™) were used.

Parental stress was assessed by the Center for Epidemiologic Studies Depression (CES-D) scale, a self-report screening tool for depressive symptoms. (35)

The CES-D contains 20 items that evaluate the frequency of depressive symptoms during the preceding week. Ratings are summed to calculate a total CES-D score, which can range from 0 to 60. A score of 16 points or above indicates frequent experience of depressive symptoms. We used a score of 7 or higher to indicate distress in parents which has been used in previous studies. For children seen in follow-up one year later, we devised a structured interview survey.

The survey was a 15-item questionnaire that measured child and parent well-being, satisfaction with services, and child's current developmental status. In the follow-up portion of this study, a total of 41 families completed these interviews.

Data analysis: Phase 1

To compare domains by controlling for age, standard scores or developmental quotients (DQ) was calculated for each assessment. DQ is calculated as the performance age equivalence divided by chronological age of the patient.

In Illinois, children eligible for Early Intervention services have their percent delay expressed as 1 minus the standard score. Children were compared on several domains including total communication skills (receptive and expressive language), adaptive skills (activities of daily living, socialization, and functional communication which were averaged into a modified adaptive skills composite), across developmental diagnostic groups, and parental stress scores. Total communication was calculated by finding the mean between the receptive and expressive language domains.

The data was analyzed using SPSS and t-tests and ANOVA were used to measure differences between groups. Statistical significance was defined by $p < 0.05$.

Findings

Patient characteristics

Data from 230 patients who were diagnosed with mixed developmental disorder, autism or global developmental delay was obtained. Table 1 describes the patient characteristics in total and by diagnostic group.

Table 1. Young children with autism, global delays or mixed developmental disorders

	Autism (n = 99)	Global developmental delay (n = 48)	Mixed developmental disorder (n=83)
Total Communication DQ	.47 ± .19 (n=83)	.52 ± .22 (n = 44)	.65 ± .20 (n =70)
Daily Living Skills DQ	.60 ± .15 (n =65)	.62 ± .19 (n=45)	.70 ± .16 (n = 62)
Socialization DQ	.46 ± .16 (n=53)	.60 ± .24 (n = 45)	.63 ± .19 (n=58)
Adaptive Behavior Composite DQ	.52 ± .14 (n =57)	.59 ± .19 (n=45)	.66 ± .15 (n=58)
Parent Stress	9.55 ± 8.30 (n = 42)	8.32 ± 6.73 (n=31)	10.02 ± 8.36 (n = 34)

In our sample, 83 patients were diagnosed with mixed developmental disorder, 99 with autism and 48 with global developmental delay. The mean age of patients was 31.8 ± 10 months and 77% were male.

The predominance of males was highest in children with autism (87%) and lowest in children with global developmental delay (65%). Children with autism were also the oldest to come to initial evaluation (36.3 ± 9.8 months) whereas children with global developmental delay came earliest (26 ± 7.8 months), and children with mixed developmental disorders were assessed at 31.8 ± 10.1 months. Evaluation outcomes are described for each group by communication, daily living skills, socialization, adaptive behavior composite, and parent stress. Children with autism scored lower on communication, daily living, socialization, and overall adaptive behavior.

Parental stress was high in all groups compared to children with mixed developmental disorders ($p<0.01$). Approximately 50% of parents across all groups reported that they experienced distress as measured by the CES-D.

Developmental status, parental stress and parental priorities

To examine the correlation between communication and adaptive behavior skills in preschool children with developmental delays, we used a bivariate regression model.

There was a linear relationship between adaptive and communicative skills. Children with slower rates in acquiring communication skills also had slower rates in acquiring adaptive skills. In children with global developmental delay, the relationship was most robust ($r = .87$), whereas in children with autism, this relationship was the weakest ($r = .50$). For all diagnostic groups, the correlation between adaptive and communicative skills was statistically significant ($p<.001$).

However, we did not find a significant correlation between communication skills and parental stress scores ($r = -.05$) or the correlation between adaptive behavior and parental stress scores ($r = -.13$).

Of all services, caregivers felt that speech therapists, occupational therapists, and developmental therapists were very helpful (56%, 51% and 49% respectively). About 12% of families rated school administrators as not helpful at all and 10% of pediatricians/family physicians as not helpful at all.

The majority of caregivers (88%) agreed that they were more knowledgeable about how to help their child learn and that they became more knowledgeable about their child's developmental strengths and weaknesses after receiving a multidisciplinary medical diagnostic assessment.

However, 39% felt that their child's developmental condition caused financial problems and 46% stated that their family had to cut back on work hours to meet their child's needs. In addition, almost 2 in 3 families (63%) noted that their priorities and goals for their child hadchanged as well.

Only 12% of caregivers rated their child's current developmental status as excellent or very good, 29% rated their child's behavior as excellent or very good, but 68% rated their child's health in general as excellent or very good. With respect to caregiver physical health, 51% of respondents rated themselves as having excellent or very good health status, 31.7% responded good and 17% responded fair or poor.

About one-third (32%) of participants reported that their mental health and peace of mind was fair or poor while 37% responded that their current supports for their children were fair or poor. In regards to caregiver stress levels over the previous 12 months, almost 3 in 5 (59%) felt that their stress level was very intense or high.

Study 2

Parent-therapist-preschool collaborative treatment model for young children with autism

In developing our treatment model, we incorporated the recommendations of the Committee on Educational Interventions for Children with Autism (5). Our program emphasized early intervention, intensive instructional programming, and intense training of parents.

We followed the expert panel's recommendations for young children with autism so that children received interventions that addressed the following six dimensions: 1) teach functional, spontaneous communication; 2) provide social skill instruction throughout the day in various settings; 3) teach play skills, including the appropriate use of toys and objects; 4) focus on cognitive goals, with programming for generalization across settings; 5) address problematic behaviors, using techniques and interventions with empirical support, such as functional analysis of behavior and reinforcement of alternative behaviors; and 6) teach academic skills keeping in mind the individual needs of each child.

To develop this comprehensive approach, the authors integrated significant aspects of The TEACCH Model (25), The Heartland Hand-in-Hand Model (36), and the Lovaas' Discrete Trial Format (22). Our approach also included utilization of The Picture Exchange Communication System (PECS) (37), Greenspan's Floor Time model (38), and the principles of applied behavior analysis and sensory integration approaches. These approaches were chosen for their individual strengths as listed in table 2.

Table 2. Strengths of the approaches selected for the integrated curriculum

TEACCH	Structured teaching, visual and physical structure
Heartland Hand in Hand	Structured teaching with comprehensive skills
Picture Exchange Communication system	Visual communication system
Greenspan's Floor Time	Socialization and pleasurable interaction
Lovaas' Discrete Trial Format	Individual skill development
Sensory Integration Approaches	Sensory "diet"
Applied Behavior Analysis	Analysis and treatment of problem behaviors

The approaches chosen for this study were selected because they address the neuropsychological profile of strengths and weaknesses often seen in individual children with autism. These patterns include: strength in responding to visual cues and in visual learning; lowered responding to auditory cues in spite of adequate hearing; poor sequential memory;

good rote learning and memory; heightened arousal levels, sensory hypo-sensitivities and hyper-sensitivities; difficulties with self regulation, including poor attention, distractibility, increased activity levels and restlessness; and difficulties playing appropriately with objects or toys, often with non-functional use of these items.

Table 3 summarizes how the intervention approach was constructed to address weaknesses and to teach to the strengths of the young child with autism.

Table 3. Intervention strategies to address the unique learning style of children with autism

Learning profile	Intervention strategies
Lowered responding to auditory cues and strength in responding to visual cues and enhanced visual learning	Combine visual supports (i.e., PECS, visual schedules, and visual cues) with verbal and motor cues to enhance understanding and learning
Poor sequential memory	Use of picture schedules to increase understanding of time, sequence, and independent functioning
Better rote learning and rote memory	Use of Structured Teaching approaches and Discrete Trial teaching methods to increase skills
Sensory integration difficulties, with heightened arousal levels, sensory hypo-sensitivities, sensory hyper-sensitivities, and shortened attention span	Use of "sensory diets" to help modulate arousal levels, use of schedules to increase predictability and decrease anxiety, and sensory modes to help with self-regulation and attention (i.e., adult provides controls to help child internalize control)
Difficulties playing appropriately with objects/toys	Use of Floor Time techniques to help expand play and decrease non-functional use of objects; inclusion of sensory play to address non-functional use of objects due to sensory seeking behaviors
Difficulties communicating functionally, at times in spite of the presence of verbal language skills	Use of PECS to enhance functional communication skills in non-verbal children and use of Social Stories and Floor Time techniques to increase functional speech

Individualized programming

To individualize programming for children, developmentally and behaviorally organized strands were developed in seven areas: 1) attention and compliance, 2) imitation, 3) communication, 4) self-help and daily living skills, 5) play and social development, 6) academic skills and 7) problematic behaviors.

To implement the program, home-based intervention for all children included developing physical structure in the home and establishing daily visual schedules and work systems.

These techniques were then used to teach the children new skills and to practice skills that had already been mastered. To individualize the program, weekly goals were established for each child in the seven areas of functioning addressed in the curriculum. Skills identified as emerging in an initial functional assessment were used to establish the treatment plan. Therapists and parents worked on the specified goals throughout the week, completing a structured format for data collection.

Parent training

Parent training consisted of 20 hours of instruction over four days, which included both didactic and "hands-on" experiences. Participation of both parents and/or caretakers was required. Parents signed a written contract to participate fully in the training, to attend all sessions, and to complete all training tasks. In the parent training sessions, parents who had successfully completed the treatment program assisted the staff with training new parents. The opportunity to interact with seasoned parents appeared to provide significant support for the new parents, reducing their anxiety and helping them become more comfortable with taking on new challenges. As parents worked cooperatively to understand and apply intervention concepts, group cohesion developed that furthered the psychological process of taking on the new roles and demands required by this collaborative treatment approach.

Specific training modules were developed (39) to assure that parents had the requisite store of information and skills to carry out the program at home and in the community and are highlighted in table 4. The focus was on increasing parental knowledge regarding different principles and approaches that they could utilize in helping their children in the home and in the community.

Table 4. Parent training modules

1. Characteristics of autism	Patterns of development, learning styles, social impairments, deficits in abstract thought and "theory of mind"
2. Communication deficits	Language development, alternative modes of communication, including augmentative devices, such as the Picture Exchange communication System (PECS)
3. Structured teaching approaches	The TEACCH Model and the expansion of techniques in the Heartland Hand in Hand Model; use of picture schedules to understand and predict events throughout the day; work systems to each new skills and practice mastered skills; the importance of structure(both physical arrangement of the environment and visual cues) to help children understand daily routines and activities
4. Applied behavior analysis	Use of ABA and discrete trial teaching to manage and prevent problem behaviors as well as to teach basic skills of attending and compliance
5. Social development	Enhancing affective development and social interaction skills, utilizing direct teaching of social skills and use of Floor Time techniques

6. Sensory regulatory difficulties	Sensory integration difficulties in autism; hypo and hyper sensitivities; problems with arousal, attention, activity level and distractibility
7. Data based approaches	Functional assessment, data collection techniques and the use of standardized tests.

Parent-therapist implemented treatment was presented to 20 young children with autism to determine whether an integrated approach, implemented by parents and therapists in the home environment, could significantly improve children's developmental outcomes and could produce learning rates that are comparable to more intensive and hence more expensive approaches. Learning rates reported by more intensive approaches were used as a benchmark to evaluate the effectiveness of the integrative treatment.

Participants: Phase 2

The treatment group included 20 children with autism, between the ages of two years and six years 11 months. Sessions were conducted in English, except for the Latino families where Spanish-speaking therapists conducted sessions in Spanish. All families resided in the city of Chicago. All participants were enrolled in Early Childhood Special Education classes in the Chicago Public Schools, receiving speech therapy and occupational therapy weekly in the school as part of their regular special education programming 10-15 hours per week. All children entering the program had been diagnosed with autism by a multidisciplinary team, using a battery of instruments with demonstrated effectiveness in the early diagnosis of autism, including the Autism Diagnostic Interview-Revised (ADI-R) and the Autism Diagnostic Observation Schedule (ADOS).

Treatment protocol

The treatment program was a relatively short, home based program divided into two phases: 1) Parent training (20 hours) and 2) Home based intervention (4 months).

Parent training

A total of 43 parents participated in the parent trainings. Of the families participating, 17 were intact families, two were divorced families (where both parents participated although living in separate homes), and one was a single mother. Parents participated in a four-day, 20-hour parent training at the Medical Center. The parent training included a combination of lectures, videos, and hands-on activities as indicated in table 4.

Treatment program

The four months of intensive intervention included three weekly visits to the home where the therapists worked with each child for 60 minutes, addressing the specific goals drafted for each area of functioning, for a total of 48 professional therapy hours. During each visit, an additional 30 minutes was dedicated to the family to address specific questions, review goals, and provide feed-back and suggestions for improvement, for a total of 24 hours of home based consultation time. The family provided an additional 10 hours of therapy for their child on a weekly basis, working on the established goals, for a total of 160 parent-directed therapy hours. Families used the structure and work system set up in their homes to teach new skills, as well as more naturalistic learning out in the community to help with maintenance and generalization of skills.

Weekly goal sheets were completed for each area of functioning every week. Thus, a total of seven goals sheets were drafted on a weekly basis, addressing the specific goal, criteria for meeting the goal, and materials/reinforcers to be used. Weekly goals had an established percentage criterion for meeting the goal, 80 to 85% success rate. In addition, before a new goal was drafted, the established goal was mastered with two or more people in two or more settings on three consecutive days of data collection. This extra criterion ensured that the skill was generalized and did not remain person or context specific.

Therapists and parents collected data on their child's progress in meeting the established goals. Therapists reviewed data sheets with the family during the 30-minute consultation period on the last day of week the therapist was scheduled to be in the home. Parents were able to ask questions and therapists provided feedback on improvement of data collection and time management. The internal data sheets (collected by both parents and therapists to monitor goals, monitor parent-directed therapy hours working on designated goals) and the daily checklists used by therapists to verify that the schedules, work system, and communication systems were in place in the home, were used to document progress and mastery of specific goals based on the criterion outlined above.

Measures outcomes phase 2

Each child was evaluated using standardized instruments, including the Psychoeducational Profile-Revised (PEP-R), (40) the Vineland Adaptive Behavior Scale (VABS), the Expressive One-Word Picture Vocabulary Test(EOWPVT), and the Peabody Picture Vocabulary Test 3rd Edition(PPVT III), as well as the functional assessment based on the curriculum strands. All testing, except for the curriculum assessment and the VABS, was performed by psychologists or doctoral students who were not involved in the autism program and had no knowledge of the child's status in the program, i.e., pre or post treatment.

All children were assessed prior to the initiation of home-based services and after the four-month intensive phase of the treatment. The results of the assessment battery, including all standardized instruments, as well as the functional assessment, served as outcome measures to determine efficacy of program and significance of improvements.

A functional assessment scale (FAS) determined the child's level of functioning across the different domains of the curriculum. This measure was administered by the child's therapist pre and post-treatment. The goal of this instrument was to determine how much progress was made in each curriculum area. This evaluation was also included in the post-treatment evaluation protocol as a measure of specific skills acquired.

Data analysis: Phase 2

The t test for correlated (dependent) samples was used to analyze the data obtained, given that the design measures subjects twice, with an intervening treatment. A two-tailed paired samples t test, at .05 significance level, was used to determine efficacy of the model and significance of the progress made in learning rate by the children in the four months of home-based treatment. The first set of analyses performed were the paired samples t tests for each subscale of the PPVT-III, EOWPVT, PEP-R, VABS, and the FAS. These tests were performed to determine whether there had been any statistical or clinical differences from baselinel to post-treatment.

Our findings

Table 5 shows the descriptive characteristics of the 20 participants and their parents. Table 6 shows that paired samples tests were performed on standardized assessments, the Psychoeducational Profile-Revised (PEP-R) and the Vineland Adaptive Behavior Scales, as well as the results of the curriculum-based functional assessment scale (FAS). The t-tests for the PPVT-III and EO-WPVT were both found to be non-significant.

Significant improvement in functional communication skills were demonstrated by increases in the Communication Domain of the Vineland Adaptive Behavior Scales, the Communication Domain of the Functional Assessment, and the Cognitive Verbal domain on the PEP-R.

Table 5. Descriptive information of participants and parents/caregivers

Subject	Gender	CA*	DA*	DQ[a]	Ethnicity	SES[b]
1	M	35	19	54.3	African-American	2
2	M	77	25	32.5	Caucasian	2
3	F	49	20	40.8	Caucasian	2
4	M	46	17	37	Caucasian	2
5	M	69	21	30.4	Hispanic	3
6	M	50	19	38	Hispanic	2
7	M	60	21	35	Asian	1
8	M	46	20	43.5	Asian	2
9	M	41	18	43.9	Asian	2
10	M	74	48	64.9	Hispanic	2
11	M	74	48	64.9	Caucasian	1
12	F	67	13	19.4	African-American	3
13	M	31	12	38.7	Caucasian	2

14	M	68	24	35.3	Caucasian	2
15	M	58	18	31	Caucasian	1
16	M	55	19	34.6	Bi-racial	2
17	M	55	18	32.7	Caucasian	2
18	F	46	20	43.5	Hispanic	3
19	M	38	22	57.9	Caucasian	2
20	M	44	14	31.8	Hispanic	3

Note. *All ages in months at Time 1 (pre-treatment).

[a]DQ: Developmental Quotient was calculated taking the developmental age over chronological age and multiplying by 100.

[b]SES: 1 = High to high-middle, 2 = Middle, 3 = Lower-middle to low.

Table 6. Developmental and social-communicative functional changes: Paired t test

	T
PEP-R scale	
Imitation	4.22***
Perception	3.02**
Fine motor	3.58**
Gross motor	3.04**
Eye-hand integration	2.74*
Cognitive performance	5.89***
Cognitive verbal	2.46*
Overall developmental score	5.19***
FAS scales	
Attention and compliance	6.59***
Verbal imitation	4.91***
Non-verbal imitation	7.38***
Receptive language skills	6.52***
Expressive Language Skills	5.84***
Play and imaginative/creative skills	4.08***
Social awareness and joint attention	2.78*
Emotions and gestures	1.93
Drawing and pre-writing skills	2.90**
Matching and categorization	5.91***
General knowledge	4.53***
Self help and daily living skills	7.15***
Problematic behaviors	2.80**
Vineland domain	
Communication skills	3.18**
Daily living skills	3.96***
Social skills	3.66**

* = $p<0.05$, ** = $p < 0.01$, *** = $p<0.001$.

Significant increases in social awareness and interaction skills were found in the Socialization Domain of the Vineland Adaptive Behavior Scales, the Imitation and Social Development domains in the Functional Assessment Scale, and the Imitation Domain in the PEP-R.

Significant improvement in school readiness skills were seen by the increases in Attending, Compliance, and Academic Domains of FAS, increases in Perception, Eye-hand integration, and Cognitive Performance Domains in the PEP-R. Independent functioning was also significantly enhanced as seen in the increases in the Daily Living Skills Domain of the Vineland Adaptive Behavior Scales and the Self-help and Daily Living Skills domain in the functional assessment.

Additionally, a large importance was placed on decreasing the likelihood of problematic behaviors. Results showed that these children successfully reduced the frequency of negative behaviors such as tantrums and aggression as indicated on the FAS. Additional feedbacks from PUENTES participants revealed that parents' sense of competence significantly increased. Lastly, the cost of this intervention for the first year was $14,000, significantly less than the current cost for 25 hour one-on-one discreet trial intervention.

Discussion

The idea that lower communications skills would be associated with lower adaptive skills was supported by our data, though this relationship was most variable amongst children with autism. Research has shown that adaptive behavior presentation in preschool children may vary and some children with autism have higher daily living skills, whereas others have not.

Our study did not find a strong association between adaptive or communicative skills and parent stress.

One explanation for this result may be a limitation in our assessment tool. The CES-D scale is used to screen for depression which means it may not be an accurate indicator or the most sensitive measure to parent stress. The CESD scale is also not specifically directed towards the child and his/her developmental challenges, but rather, the parent's overall mood and feelings. Therefore, other variables in parents' lives such as occupation and finances, may have influenced their responses to the survey. One of the factors that may contribute to family stress is delay in receiving school services. Our study demonstrated that home-based interventions would increase manageability at school. Of concern is that a large number of families reported that school administrators and teachers were not as helpful as habilitation therapists and developmental pediatricians.

The collaborative parent-therapist implemented treatment program described in this paper produced dramatic child change data in a very short period of time. Children who participated in the treatment program showed dramatic increases in their skills in all core areas of functioning.

Statistically significant increases were found in their functional communication skills, social development skills, school readiness skills, and independent functioning. In addition, significant decreases were observed in the very challenging problematic behaviors that tend to interfere with their ability to learn and interact successfully with others.

Clearly, defining a treatment approach that can be implemented largely by families and which leads to dramatic developmental growth in children with autism is a significant contribution to our armamentarium to address the barriers to preschool services. Further research is needed to determine whether these gains can be maintained, and to assess the relative contribution of various treatment aspects.

It is of paramount importance that comprehensive treatment programs for young children with autism be developed, with adequate outcome measures to determine efficacy.

These programs must provide adequate intensity without overburdening the family economically or emotionally.

Our treatment model shows promise for meeting these needs. By providing an integrative, comprehensive program, that focuses both on the parent and the child, we found that children and their parents were able to gain the skills and understanding needed to create the necessary bridges for coping , learning, and interacting with their environment as they make the transition to school-based services.

Acknowledgments

Supported in part by

HRSA – Department of Health and Human ServicesT73 MC11047*Leadership Education in Neurodevelopmental and Related Disorders Training Program (LEND);* NIH/NICHD P30 HD054275 *JP Kennedy* I*ntellectual and Developmental Disabilities Research Center (IDDRC),*NIH Pritzker Medical Scientist Training Grant, the Grant Healthcare, McDonald and Irving Harris Foundations. Additional thanks to the Illinois Autism Project . Special thanks to N Schwartz, Jennifer Park, L Gray, and B Andrews.

K Vanderploeg Booth, K Acharya, P Northrup, B Kniaz , P Smith, and A Berger. Richard Zur provided invaluable statistical consultation. Special thanks to Megan DiQuattro and Brandon Kopald for data collection . We gratefully acknowledge the participants and their families. This chapter was presented in part at the American Academy of Cerebral Palsy and Developmental Medicine (AACPDM) meeting in Vancouver in 2007 and at the International Meeting for Autism Research (IMFAR) meeting in Chicago in 2009.

References

[1] Autism and Developmental Disabilities Monitoring Network Surveillance Year 2002 Principal Investigators; Centers for Disease and Control and Prevention. Prevalence of autism spectrum disorders – autism and developmental disabilities monitoring network, 14 sites, United States, 2002. MMWR Surveill Summ 2007;56:12-28.

[2] Mandell DS, Novak MM, Zubritsky CD. Factors associated with age of diagnosis among children with autism spectrum disorders. Pediatrics 2005;116(6):1480-6.

[3] Newschaffer CJ, Croen LA, Daniels J, Giarelli E, Grether JK, Levy SE, Mandell DS, Miller LA, Pinto-Martin J, Reaven J, Reynolds AM, Rice CE, Schendel D, Windham GC. The epidemiology of autism spectrum disorders. Annu. Rev. Public Health 2007;28:235-58.

[4] Fombonne E. Epidemiology of pervasive developmental disorders. Pediatr. Res. 2009;65(6):591-8.

[5] Martínez-Pedraza Fde L, Carter AS. Autism spectrum disorders in young children. Child Adolesc. Psychiatr. Clin N. Am. 2009;18(3):645-63.

[6] National Research Council Committee on Educational Interventions for Children with Autism. Educating children with autism. Washington DC: Natl. Acad. Press, 2001.

[7] Johnson CP, Myers SM; American Academy of Pediatrics Council on Children With Disabilities. Identification and evaluation of children with autism spectrum disorders. Pediatrics 2007;120(5):1183-215.
[8] Myers SM, Johnson CP; American Academy of Pediatrics Council on Children With Disabilities. Management of children with autism spectrum disorders. Pediatrics 2007;120(5):1162-82.
[9] Anders TF, Gardner SE. Professional-Parent Collaboration - the M.I.N.D. institute model. In: Ozonoff S, Rogers SJ, Hendren RL, eds. Autism spectrum disorders - a research review for practitioners (pp. 227-238). Washington, DC: Am. Psychiatr. Publ, 2003.
[10] Renty J, Roeyers H. Satisfaction with formal support and education for children with autism spectrum disorder: the voices of the parents. Child Care Health Dev. 2006;32(3):371-85.
[11] Gray LA, Msall ER, Msall ME. Communicating about autism. Decreasing fears and stresses through parent-professional partnerships. Infants Young Child 2008; 21:256-71.
[12] Stahmer AC. The basic structure of community early intervention programs for children with autism: provider descriptions. J. Autism Dev. Disord. 2007;37(7):1344-54.
[13] Rogers SJ. Neuropsychology of autism in young children and its implications for early intervention. Ment. Retard Dev. Disabil. Res. Rev. 1998;4(2):104-12.
[14] Rogers SJ, Vismara LA. Evidence-based comprehensive treatments for early autism. J. Clin. Child Adolesc. Psychol. 2008;37(1):8-38.
[15] Johnson CP. Recognition of autism before age 2 years. Pediatr. Rev. 2008;29(3):86-96.
[16] Msall ME. Establishing a translational science for autistic spectrum disorders for children and their families: Optimizing function, participation, and well-being. J. Pediatr. 2009;154:319-21.
[17] Tarkan L. Autism Therapy is Called Effective, but Rare. The New York Times on the Web. Accessed June 10, 2009. http://www.wrightslaw.com/news/2002/jaynes.tarkan.nytimes.htm
[18] Marcus LM, Rubin JS, Rubin MA. Benefit-cost analysis and autism services: a response to Jacobson and Mulick. J. Autism Dev. Disord. 2000;30(6):595-8.
[19] Spreckley M, Boyd R. Efficacy of applied behavioral intervention in preschool children with autism for improving cognitive, language, and adaptive behavior: A systematic review and meta-analysis. J. Pediatr. 2009;154:338-44.
[20] Ospina MB, Krebs Seida J, Clark B, Karkhaneh M, Hartling L, Tjosvold L, Vandermeer B, Smith V. Behavioural and developmental interventions for autism spectrum disorder: a clinical systematic review. PLoS ONE 2008;3(11):e3755.
[21] Ben Itzchak E, Lahat E, Burgin R, Zachor AD. Cognitive, behavior and intervention outcome in young children with autism. Res. Dev. Disabil. 2008;29(5):447-58.
[22] McEachin JJ, Smith T, Lovaas OI. Long-term outcome for children with autism who received early intensive behavioral treatment. Am. J. Ment. Retard 1993;97(4):359-72.
[23] Howlin P, Magiati I, Charman T. Systematic review of early intensive behavioral interventions for children with autism. Am. J. Intellect. Dev. Disabil. 2009;114(1):23-41.
[24] Reichow B, Wolery M. Comprehensive synthesis of early intensive behavioral interventions for young children with autism based on the UCLA young autism project model. J. Autism Dev. Disord. 2009;39(1):23-41.
[25] Schopler E. Implementation of the TEACCH Philosophy. In: Cohen DJ, Volkmar FR, eds. Handbook of autism and pervasive developmental disorders, 2nd ed. New York: Wiley, 1997:767-95.
[26] Preston D, Carter M. A Review of the Efficacy of the Picture Exchange Communication System Intervention. J. Autism Dev. Disord. 2009 Jun 3. (Epub ahead of print)
[27] Prizant BM, Wetherby AM. Understanding the continuum of discrete-trial traditional behavioral to social-pragmatic developmental approaches in communication enhancement for young children with autism/PDD. Semin Speech Lang 1998;19(4):329-52.
[28] Howard JS, Sparkman CR, Cohen HG, Green G, Stanislaw H. A comparison of intensive behavior analytic and eclectic treatments for young children with autism. Res. Dev. Disabil. 2005;26(4):359-83.
[29] Magiati I, Charman T, Howlin P. A two-year prospective follow-up study of community-based early intensive behavioural intervention and specialist nursery provision for children with autism spectrum disorders. J. Child Psychol. Psychiatry 2007;48(8):803-12.
[30] Rickards AL, Walstab JE, Wright-Rossi RA, Simpson J, Reddihough DS. A randomized, controlled

trial of a home-based intervention program for children with autism and developmental delay. J. Dev. Behav. Pediatr. 2007;28(4):308-16.

[31] Stone WL, Ousley OY, Hepburn SL, Hogan KL, Brown CS. Patterns of adaptive behavior in very young children with autism. Am. J. Ment. Retard 1999;104(2):187-99.

[32] Perry A, Flanagan HE, Dunn Geier J, Freeman NL. Brief report: the Vineland Adaptive Behavior Scales in young children with autism spectrum disorders at different cognitive levels. J. Autism Dev. Disord 2009;39(7):1066-78.

[33] Anderson DK, Oti RS, Lord C, Welch K. Patterns of Growth in Adaptive Social Abilities Among Children with Autism Spectrum Disorders. J. Abnorm Child Psychol. 2009 37:1019-34

[34] Braddock D, Hemp R, Rizzolo, MC. The state of the states in developmental disabilities: 2008. Washington, DC: Am. Assoc. Intellect Dev. Disabil., 2009.

[35] Radloff LS. The CES-D Scale: A self-report depression scale for research in the general population. Applied Psychol. Measure 1977;1(3):385-401

[36] Heartland Training Model for Teaching Students with Autism. Accessed June 10, 2009. http://www.aea267.k12.ia.us/

[37] Bondy A, Frost L. The picture exchange communication system. Semin. Speech Lang. 1998;19(4):373-88.

[38] Wieder S, Greenspan SI. Climbing the symbolic ladder in the DIR model through floor time/interactive play. Autism 2003;7(4):425-35.

[39] Nanclares V. Program evaluation: An analysis of the PUENTES intensive home-based treatment program for young children with autism. Dissertation Abstracts Intl. Section B. Sci. Engineering 2004; 65 (6-B):3173.

[40] Schopler E, Reichler RJ, Bashford A, Lansing M, Marus L. Individualized Assessment and Treatment for Autistic and Developmentally Disabled Children. Vol. I: Psychoeducational Profile-Revised (PEP-R). Baltimore, MD: Univ Park Press, 1990.

In: Understanding Autism Spectrum Disorder
Editors: Ditza A Zachor and Joav Merrick

ISBN: 978-1-62081-353-9

Chapter 8

Parent-professional reporting of symptomatology and level of functioning in autism: Complementary perspectives

Cory Shulman[1]*, Sigal Tidhar-Paz,[2] and Charles Greenbaum[3]

[1]School of Social Work, Hebrew University of Jerusalem, Jerusalem, Israel [2]Department of Psychology, Haifa University, Haifa

[3]Department of Psychology, Faculty of Social Sciences, Hebrew University of Jerusalem, Jerusalem, Israel

Abstract

Parents are an integral part in the diagnosis and assessment of their children. This collaboration is important in the diagnostic assessment of children with autism, as parents know their child across various contexts and over time. In the present research, diagnostic characteristics and language skills assessed through parental reports and clinical testing of young children with autism were compared. Studying discrepancies, which emerge between parental reporting and clinical assessments may assist in understanding different perspectives regarding the child. Despite expected discordance, a high degree of agreement was found between information received from parents and clinical testing, replicating results from previous studies. In cases in which parents and professionals did not agree, parents tended to describe their children's language skills as more developed than the results from clinical testing indicated. A possible explanation for this is parents base their assessment of their child's language skills on generalized contexts, whereas professionals assess children in the specific context of an evaluation. Alternatively parents may be less objective in evaluating their child's abilities. The degree of agreement concerning the children's language skills was found to be related to the

* Correspondence: Cory Shulman, PhD, Hebrew University of Jerusalem, School of Social Work, Mount Scopus, IL-91905 Jerusalem, Israel. E-mail: mscory@mscc.huji.ac.il

children's mental age, with a higher degree of agreement in children with higher mental ages, while no such correlations emerged in the assessment of autism symptomotology. Future research should focus of the meaning of differences between informants in an attempt to understand the manner in which those involved in diagnosing autism can use information from various informants to establish appropriate intervention programs.

Introduction

It is accepted practice to include information from multiple sources in establishing a diagnosis of an autism spectrum disorder (1). Since early diagnosis has proven to be important, an effort has been made to diagnose autism and related disorders (autism spectrum disorders – ASD) as early as possible, although at young ages behavioral and developmental characteristics among various developmental disabilities overlap, making diagnostic ascertainment particularly challenging. Diagnosis of an ASD often involves many professionals, including those from the health and educational systems and as Achenbach, McConaughy and Howell (2) revealed in a meta-analysis of 119 studies, informants (e.g., parents, children, teachers) rate social, emotional and behavioral development differently. Informant discrepancies have been found in different methods of assessment (rating scales, questionnaires, and interviews) and in different clinical populations studied, such as ADHD (3), OCD, anxiety (4) and PDD (5). The importance of studying informant discrepancies cannot be overestimated since there is still no single accepted method for assessing child psychopathology. Thus, diagnosis and evaluation must incorporate information from many sources in order to get as comprehensive and valid a profile as possible, on which intervention decisions are based.

Recent research suggests that informant discrepancies may relate to critical facets of parent, child and family variables (6) or the result of process factors (i.e., components of the interaction between medical practice and patient or in this case parent behavior). A number of studies have attempted to identify factors influencing discrepancies among informants, but no theoretically relevant rationale has been provided to explain the differences which emerge from multiple informants and as a result, research has not been conducted to explain the processes involved (7-9).

The present study was undertaken as an initial step in understanding the implications of the discrepancies between parental reporting and clinical assessment of the autistic symptoms and language abilities of young children with autism. This is particularly important in the diagnosis of autism, a neurodevelopmental disability, characterized by impairments in social and communicative development and by restricted and repetitive behaviors. Because the assumption is that the underlying dysfunction has to do with qualitative deficits in communication and social abilities, professionals have to acquire information about the quality of the child's reciprocal interactions, either through the clinician's own experience with the child or from reports from the parents or both (1).

Parent-professional relationship

The difficulty in accurately diagnosing the disorder can add tension to the parent-professional relationship. Since there is no biological test for autism, autism is diagnosed when substantial behavioral indicators are present, and when there is no evidence for an alternative diagnosis. Although parents commonly suspect their child's condition before the official diagnosis is made, they typically come to the diagnostic situation hoping that their fears will not be confirmed by the professional's diagnosis. Since their perceptions of their child may be different from those of professionals, there is a tendency to think that one must be right. One of the goals of the present research is to investigate these differences and try to understand how they can inform us.

Parent perspectives are subjective, but yet important and relevant. The term 'congruence' refers to the degree of correspondence or agreement between individuals' judgments and not to the accuracy of those judgments. If information from various sources agrees, the credibility of that information is enhanced. When congruence is low, it can be informative and it is important to examine possible reasons for the discrepancies (10). In one of the initial attempts to understand these differences, Stone and Rosenbaum (11) compared the perceptions of parents of children with autism to the perceptions of professionals, who were specialists in autism. Parents were found to harbor misconceptions regarding cognitive, developmental and emotional features of autism, as they tended to view autistic individuals as less cognitively impaired. Despite these differences information from the parents regarding their child's development has potential value in the early diagnosis of autism and assessment of the child.

Parental reporting

The idea of using parents as a source of data, especially in pediatric clinical practice, is not new. Pediatricians rely on parents to provide a considerable portion of the data they use to diagnose children's illnesses. The information obtained from parents serves as a useful and important complement to medical tests and procedures. Nowadays, parents are active participants in their child's assessment, reflecting professionals' belief that the best assessment is made by synthesizing the information collected from multiple sources.

The information gathered from parents is especially important for the assessment of infants and young children who are not always cooperative in the assessment process (10, 12, 13).Because of their developmental status, there are many factors that might influence their performance during formal testing such as fatigue or lack of familiarity with the examiner. Another advantage of using parent reports relates to the unique perspectives parents offer relating their child's personality and their child's developmental history and difficulties (6,10). In addition to the relevance of parent reports to their children's assessment process, parent reports have treatment relevance, reflecting parental attitudes and perceptions of the child's behavior.

The parent professional collaboration during assessment can help to focus the parent's attention on age-appropriate behaviors (14). Finally, parental estimations regarding specific behaviors can establish a mutual base for discussions between parents and professionals. When parents take an active part in the assessment process, they feel that their observations are valuable and their concerns about their child's development are being addressed (15).

Parental versus professional reporting

Several studies reported that although parents can provide clinically useful information, their estimations tend to be higher than those of professionals. For example, Stiles (15) reviewed 24 studies and found that in 18 of them (75%), parents estimates where higher than those of professionals. Dinnebeil and Rule (10) reviewed 23 studies regarding comparisons between parent estimates and professionals assessments. Typically developing children and those with developmental delays, aged 0-6 years were assessed, and despite strong positive correlations between parental and professional judgments, the parents' estimates of their children's abilities were about 3.6 months higher than professionals' estimations of the same abilities.

Possible explanations for the descrepancies included that parental judgments are based on broader contexts than the context in which the professionals assess the children and professionals may underestimate children's abilities through the use of standardized tests that limit the manner of data taking. Dspite descrepencies, overall high positive correlations were found between parental reports and professionals assessments across studies. The highest correlations were found when the different observers judged the same behaviors, in the same context, with the same data collection systems. Bryne, Backman and Smith (14) examined 138 children, from one year of age to six and a half years, using the Minnesota Child Development Inventory (MCDI) High correlations were found between parents and professionals regarding the developmental status of preschoolers, but significantly poorer correlations regarding the developmental status of infants emerged. Miller et al (16) compared mothers' and professionals' assessments of 53 children with developmental delays. Generally, high correlation was found, although over the different developmental areas, mothers estimated the children as developmentally higher than the professionals. IQ was found to be the best predictor for assessments agreements. Voelker et al (17) studied congruence of adaptive functioning in low functioning children of parental reporting and results from professional assessments and found less agreement between teacher and parents than had been reported for higher functioning children. A possible explanation may be that the lower functioning the child is the more difficult it is to assess their level of functioning accurately as found in the differences which emerged between congruence studies of infants and those of preschool aged children. Parental reports regarding children from special populations can be summarized by saying that there is a correlation between parental estimates of their children's behaviors and those of the professionals. At the same time, when specific characteristics of the disabilities and behaviors are being estimated in greater depth there are some differences. Therefore, when congruence is being checked between parent reports and professionals' assessments, it is important to refer to the characteristics of the disabilities and to the specific characteristics of the behaviors being assessed.

Autism is a neurological, developmental disorder. Unlike congruence studies with other populations, there is lack of studies which investigate degrees of agreement between parents and professionals in assessing children with autism. This lack is surprising especially in the light of the integral role parents of children with autism take in the diagnostic process of their children (1,13). In a study of children ages 4 to 6 with Pervasive Developmental Disorder (PDD) parent and teachers' assessments where compared. The children were assessed on their diagnostic and adaptive behavior skills. The researchers used the 'Autism Behavior Checklist' (ABC) (18) as a diagnostic measure and the 'Vineland Adaptive Behavior' (VABS) (5) to assess the children's adaptive behaviors. They found that there was relatively good agreement between the parents and the teachers regarding the children's level of adaptive functioning, although teachers tended to rate the children a bit higher than the parents. In contrast, there was low congruence regarding behaviors connected to the diagnosis of autism on the ABC. The suggested explanation for higher estimation of the teachers may be that they have a lower threshold than parents in deciding whether an adaptive behavior is present or not, as a result of either the length of time they know the children or their commitment to children with special needs. The teachers also have more opportunities to observe the children's behaviors assessed by the VABS. The school environment is usually more structured than home and has more time, ability and stimuli resources to observe the adaptive abilities of the children. On the other hand, because of the differences in expectations and structure between home and school, ASD children may well exhibit more ASD behaviors and less adaptive skills at home than at school.

Cross informant inconsistency

Assessing young children with autism presents a professional challenge. The uneven pattern of developmental skills makes it difficult to assess the intellectual abilities of the young child, with low functioning, younger children with autism presenting an even greater challenge in assessment.

Reliance on multiple informants for assessment of adaptive behavior is a valuable and often necessary alternative to traditional assessment (17). Obtaining information from informants who know the child well, such as parents provides a rich source of data on the abilities that the child displays in various contexts. Yet, there is a problem with cross-informant inconsistency.For example, only modest correlations have been observed between third party ratings and child behavior which can also be inconsistent over context (15).

Mata-analysis (2) found the highest congruence among ratings of children's behavior and emotional problems among raters who played a similar role in the child's life such as Teacher X Teacher comparison (Pearson r = .60). Substantially lower agreement was noted for raters with different roles with respect to the child, such as Parent X Teacher (Pearson r = .28).

Reviews of parent/.teacher agreement in ratings of developmental status of young children with disabilities (17) and on measures of adaptive behavior have tended to find higher rates of agreement than those reported for problem behaviors. Likewise, methodological issues, statistical issues, and procedural issues (e.g., which tests or measurements are used in order to decide on differences) have contributed to the inconsistencies in the findings. When parent/professional disagreements have been reportedoften parents report greater skills than did professionals.

The Vineland Adaptive Behavior Scales have been used in assessing parental evaluations of levels of adaptive functioning (5, 17). Parent and teacher ratings on the instrument were highly correlated indicating close agreement on relative ranking of the children, however the teachers systematically rated the children as more skilled that the parents did. Interrater discrepancies reported for children may be significant enough to have an impact on placement and programming decisions.

Taking advantage of multiple sources of information for making decisions about program planning is recommended (19), but this advice presumes good interrater reliability for the measures used and some appropriate means for evaluation of any systematic sources of disagreement that may occur. Discrepancies between ratings may reflect unreliability or lack of comparability of measure/s, rater bias, or genuine differences in the child's behavior across contexts.

Patterns of discrepancies must be examined further inorder to understand the implications of both agrees of agreement and discrepancies. Therefore, the present study examines patterns of agreement and disagreement in parental reporting and results of professional testing of young children with ASD, in order to further investigate possible sources of cross-informant discrepancies in autism symptomology and developmental/adaptive abilities.

Purpose

The main purpose of this study was to learn more about different information obtained from various sources and the possible contexts for attaining wider diagnostic and developmental aspects concerning children with autism. Thus, it is important to include information received from parental reports in addition to that received from professionals' assessments of the children,and to relate to the agreement level between the two informants. Another purpose of this study was to improve the proficiency of the early assessment of children with autism. Early assessment is a necessary component for reaching better decisions regarding appropriate placement, appropriate strategies for intervention and the appropriate manner in which to establish a parent-professionla collaboration. This study deals with the assessment of young children with ASD (ages 3-6 years), including the diagnosis of autism and the assessment of the children's general developmental level, specifically focusing on level of language skills, which has been identified as an outcome measure in ASD. Assessing younger children enables diagnostic ascertainment of autism and its associated difficulties, which in turn enables appropriate placement and treatment at an early stage. At the same time, establishing a diagnosis at younger ages is more complicated than diagnostic ascertainment is at older ages, because of the similarities between early behavioral characters of autism and normal behavioral characters or of other disabilities. Diagnosis at early ages is also more complicated because not all the diagnostic characteristics of autism are evident yet. Thus, this study which also focuses on assessing young children at the critical developmental age (3-6 years) can contribute to the the process of assessment during this key stage of development of the diagnostic symptoms related to ASD.

Thus, the study of the assessment process through the investigation of degrees of agreement between parents and professionals can also lend further information about the manifestations of autism at earlier ages. Research in the assessment of young children with autism is essential because of the lack of consensus which still exists regarding the nature of the disability and the resulting difficulties inherent in the establishment of a diagnosis of autism (1). Autism has no clear biological base, and therefore the diagnosis continues to be based on behavioral indicators (5). This type of assessment potentially evokes disagreements among different assessors regarding the presence or absence of the unique characteristics, as well as the quality of their presentation. Thus, it is important to research the levels of agreement between parents and professionals, two of the central sources of information in the assessment process. Conclusions regarding the differences between parental reports and the results form professionals' assessments can also contribute to the relationship between the two, as the assessment process is the first phase of the collaboration between parents and professionals. It is important that they share the same language right from the beginning which will allow the relationship to grow between them.

As mentioned, there are studies that showed that assessment tools using parent reports are valid tools (14,16, 18). Also, there are studies that compared parents' reports regarding their children's behavjor to the reports by those same children's teachers (5), but as yet, there is no research comparing parental reports of children with autism and clinical assessments of these children. Thus, the purpose of the current research is not to validate the tools based on parent reports, because the tools that were used in the research are standardized and have high validity and reliability, but rather, the purpose is to compare assessments of children with autism that were based on two different perspectives – the parents' and the professionals'- regarding the diagnostic characteristics of autism and the children's developmental language skills.

Our study

The sample consisted of 30 children (27 boys, 3 girls) ranging in age from 2 year 11 months to 5 years 10 months (M = 53.48; SD = 8.15; in months). There was an overrepresentation of males in this sample reflecting the 4-6:1 ratio of males to females with autism as reported in the literature (1). All the children met the diagnostic criteria for autism according to thc Diagnostic Statistical Manual (20) and the International Classification of Diseases (21), as ascertained by the Autism Diagnostic Observation Schedule (ADOS: 22) and the Autism Diagnostic Interview-Revised (ADI-R: 23). It is important to note that all the children met diagnostic criteria for autism on both the ADOS and the ADI-R. Since we were interested in parental reporting and wanted to control for language comprehension of the the parents, we included only families who were native Hebrew speakers.Likewise, all the children were living at home with their biological parents and their parents were their primary caregivers. Children with other developmental syndromes (e.g., Noonan syndrome, fragile X) or neurological conditions (e.g., epilepsy, deafness) were excluded.

Children with unspecified cognitive impairment were included. Intellectual abilities were assessed through standardized developmental assessment. The children were enrolled in special preschool/kindergarten programs for children with autism in Jerusalem, Israel.

Table 1. Sample characteristics

	Mean	Standard Deviation	Range
Chronological age (in months)	53.48	8.15	35-70
Mental age (in months)	31.86	12.01	12.75-57.75
Maternal age (in years)	35	4.32	28-43
Paternal age (in years)	37.3	4.65	29-44
Number of children in family	2.62	1.15	1-6
Birth order	.99	.14	1-5
Gender (males/females)	27 / 3		

Instruments

Instruments of direct clinical assessment of child (professional measures)

Autism Diagnostic Observation Schedule (ADOS) (22): The ADOS is a clinical scale, which consists of standard situations (presses) that allow the examiner to observe the occurrence or non-occurrence of behaviors associated with the diagnosis of autism. The structured activities and materials are intended to stimulate communication, social interaction, play and imaginative use of materials for individuals suspected of having autism or other pervasive developmental disorders. Overall ratings are made which arethen be used to formulate a diagnosis.

Mullen Scales of Early Learning (MSEL) (24): The Mullen Scales of Early Learning are a comprehensive scale of developmental domains which assess a young child's learning abilities and patterns. The scale measures nonverbal and verbal skills, documenting both receptive and expressive abilities in each domain. The full Mullen scales include tasks appropriate for assessing skills from birth to six years of age.

Instruments of informant information (parental measures)

Autism Diagnostic Interview - Revised (ADI-R) (23): The ADI-R, a semi-structured interview, is administered to the child's primary caregiver in an attempt to obtain "detailed descriptions of behaviors necessary for a differential diagnosis of pervasive developmental diagnosis (PDD) and especially for the diagnosis of autism" (p. 5). The interview focuses on key diagnostic features concerned with deviance in reciprocal social interactions, language and communication, and play skills, and restrictive, repetitive and stereotyped behaviors and interests specified in ICD-10 and DSM-IV. The ADI-R is an investigator-based interview in which it is necessary to obtain detailed descriptions of the child's actual behavior which are then coded and used in order to establish a diagnosis.

Vineland Adaptive Behavior Scales (VABS) (25): The Vineland Adaptive Behavior Scales, containing 297 items that assess four domains of functioning from birth to adulthood, do not require direct administration of tasks to an individual, but instead is based on the report of a respondent who is familiar with the individual's behavior in the domains of communication, daily living skills, socialization abilities and motor skills (for children 6 and under). The Vineland Adaptive Behavior Scales are norm referenced. and have been used and specifically tested with children diagnosed with autism.

Sequenced Inventory of Communication Development (SICD) (26): The Sequenced Inventory of Communication Development was developed to assess the processes that contribute to an individual's communicative interaction with the environment. There are two major scales evaluating receptive and expressive abilities but within each scale the tasks reflect a communication model which includes the child's awareness of communication, ability to discriminate and to understand. The assessment involves motor, vocal and verbal behaviors as well as imitation and initiation behaviors.

Procedure

After receiving permission from the Ministries of Health,and Education, a letter was sent to the parents of the children in the special autism programs, explaining the research and asking permission to contact them about the participation of their children in the research. After obtaining informed consent, diagnostic ascertainment was accomplished through the interviewing of the parents with the ADI-R. At the same time the other interview instruments were administered at the same time, including the Vineland Adaptive Behavior Scales and the Sequenced Inventory of Communication Development. The decision to include the interview instruments at this state was based on parental time constraintsThe child was then assessed with the ADOS, SICD and Mullen.

Findings

Overall agreement among professionals and parents was estimated using both correlational analyses and means comparisons. Following the example in the Szatmari et al (5) and Voelker et al (17) studies, the data were analyzed using Pearson correlations to estimate degree of agreement and then analyzed using paired ttests to determine whether disagreement was random or systematic.

The agreement between parental reporting of autism symptomotology and the results of clinical testing was calculated by comparing the scores of the selected items from the Autism Diagnostic Interview – Revised (ADI-R; 23) for the parental coding and from the Autism Diagnostic Observation Schedule (ADOS) (22).

It is important to remember that the purpose of calculating the correlations between the parental reporting on the ADI-R and the clinical results from the ADOS was not in order to test interrater reliability, but rather in order to assess the degree of agreement between the parental reporting and the results obtained by the professional in clinical assessment. The degree of agreement between the overall ADI and the ADOS scores was 41.34 (SD=15.74). The correlation between the overall score of autism symptomotology as reported by parents and as scored by professionals was high, as expected ($r=.63$, $p<.01$).

The agreement between parental reporting of language skills and the results of clinical testing was calculated by comparing the coding of selected items from the Vineland Adaptive Behavior Scales – Communication and Socialization Scales for the parental coding and from selected items from the Mullen Scales of Early Learning (24) and from the Sequenced Inventory of Communication Development (SICD-R) (26). The degree of agreement between the SICD and the MSEL scores was 85.62 (SD=13.04).

The correlation between overall scores of language and communication skills as reported by parents on the Vineland Adaptive Behavior Scales and as observed amd coded by professionals on the Mullen Scales of Early Learning and the Sequenced Inventory of Communication Development was significantly higher ($r = .81$, $p<.001$) than that reported for autism symptomotology.

Looking into possible variables which affected these results, two background factors were analyzed. No significant effects were found in the degree of agreement between the parents who had more parenting experience, which was measured by the number of children in the family, or between the parents with more knowledge of developmental milestones measured by a questionnaire regarding typical development.

Table 2. Items: Autism symptomatology

ADOS-Clinical Assessment with Psychologist	ADI-R Interview with Parents
Language and Communication	
Vocalization Directed to Others A2	Social Chat 16
Pointing A3	Pointing 30
Use of Other's Body to Communicate A4	Use of other's body to communicate 11
Gestures A5	Gestures 31
Intonation A6	Intonation 26
Immediate Echolalia A7	Immediate Echolalia 17
Stereotyped Utterances A8	Stereotyped Utterances 18
Reciprocal Social Interaction	
Eye contact B1	Eye contact 42
Social smile B7	Social smile 43
Directs facial expression to others B8	Range of facial expressions for communication 52
Giving B10	Sharing 46
Showing B11	Showing and directing attention 45
Quality of Social Overtures B16	Quality of social overtures 51
Play	Play
Imagination and creativity C2	Imagination and creativity 63
Behavior	Behavior
Repetitive behavior D1	Repetitive behavior 71
Sensory interests D3	Sensory interests 77
Hand and finger mannerisms D4	Hand and finger mannerisms 81/84

Table 3. Parallel items for parent reporting and clinical assessment – language abilities

SICD - Psychologist	Vineland - Parents
Receptive language	
4 Response to noise out of sight	1c Orients head to noise
5 Response to familiar/unfamiliar voice	2s Responds to examiner/parent's voice
6b Response to "come to me"	5c Extends arms when responds to "come here".
9 Response to negative intonation "Don't touch"	6c Understands the meaning of "No"
10 Responds to direction "give X to me"	12c Executed instructions with object and with action
13 Points to at least 5 body parts	23c Points to body parts
23 Understands big / little	30c Identifies which of two objects not present is bigger
Number of words child understands	Number of words the child understands

SICD - Psychologist	Vineland - Parents
Expressive language	
11 Imitation of sounds and words	7cSpontaneous imitation of words and sounds
33 Expresses preference when asked	18c Expresses preference (e.g., "What do you want to play with?" when presented with various toys
Says name when asked	Says name when asked
Number of words the child says	Number of words that the child says

Table 4. Degrees of agreement by participant: Autism symptoms/language skills

Subject Number	Agreement between ADI and ADOS items (%)	Agreement between VABS and SICD/MSEL items (%)
1	29%	64%
2	44%	90%
3	71%	82%
4	29%	90%
5	47%	75%
6	29%	100%
7	29%	90%
8	24%	67%
9	41%	100%
10	18%	100%
11	38%	100%
12	41%	100%
13	65%	100%
14	79%	91%
15	35%	91%
16	59%	100%
Subject Number	Agreement between ADI and ADOS items (%)	Agreement between VABS and SICD/MSEL items (%)
17	47%	60%
18	47%	73%
19	24%	82%
20	38%	75%
21	12%	90%
22	43%	100%
23	47%	80%
24	53%	91%
25	59%	100%
26	47%	64%
27	47%	80%
28	41%	70%
29	24%	80%
30	29%	90%

Discussion

The focus of the present study was the degree of agreement between results obtained from professional assessments and information obtained from parent reports regarding autism symptoms and language abilities of young children with autism. These areas were chosen because of their centrality for diagnosis and for subsequent decisions regarding intervention and servicing. The degree of agreement between the manner in which parents and professionals viewed the presence or absence of autism symptomotoplogy was rated through the use of acknowledged diagnostic assessments (e.g., ADI-R for parental reports and ADOS for clinical assessment) and the degree of agreement between parental assessment of their children's language and communication skills was assessed using the Vineland Adaptive Behavior Scales while the clinical assessment of language and communication abilities was assessed through selected items from the SICD and the MSEL developmental tests. In accordance with previous findings (5,11) there were high degrees of agreement between parents and professionals. In those cases in which there were disagreements between parents' and professionals' assessments, parents tended to report the children's language skills as less pathological than the level which emerged from the professional testing.

A contrasting picture emerged, contrary to our hypothesis regarding degrees of agreement between the parents and the professional with respect to the children's diagnostic characteristics, wherein there were no significant differences between the informants. When there were disagreements regarding specific items, one third of the parents reported their children's autism symptoms as less pathological compared to the professionals, and one third reported a tendency towards more pathology. Regarding the comparison between parental report and results fm professional assessment in the area of language skills, for those children with a high degree of agreement between the parental reporting and professional results from clinical testing regarding language skills, a significant correlation emerged between mental age and language abilities. No such correlation emerged between the mental age and the children's diagnostic characteristics among the children for whom there was not a high degree of agreement between the parents and the professionals. It appears that level of functioning is a more salient variable than chronological age when looking at degree of agreement between parents and professionals in both autism symptoms and language abilities.

The degree of agreement between parents' reports and professionals' assessments was not found to be related to the children's chronological age in this study. Likewise, degree of agreement between parent reports and professional assessments was not found to correlate with parents experience or with their knowledge of developmental milestones in childhood. This corresponds to results from previous studies which reported that directly supplying parents with information about developmental milestones was not helpful in achieving higher degrees of agreement (27). On the contrary, the researchers caution that attempting to teach parents developmental milestones, by confronting them with the discrepancies with professionals may lead to informants feeling pressured to provide ratings with are concordant with those of other informants, and as a result, important information may be lost (28). It is important to remember that it is possible that the discrepancies reflect valid differences between the sources of information available to the parents and to the professionals. Differences between informants may also develop as a result of differing degrees of objectivity that they bring to the assessment process (11), and in different expectations from the child (16) and not necessarily from differences in professional knowledge and/or prior experience. Since the information obtained from the various sources is not identical, the best assessment should include information gathered from different informants, including from parents, proessionlas and from reports and from direct assessment (11). This provides additional support to claim that parents of young children with autism should be included in the assessment of their children.

Degree of agreement was the term chosen for this research but the findings reported here are similar to those reported in other studies which studied similar phenomenon under other names, such as level of agreement among informants, informant discrepancies, correspondence among ratings, concordance or discordance among informants. Informant discrepancies have been found in virtually every method of clinical assessment that researchers and practitioners use to assess abnormalities in children (5). In this study the term 'degree of agreement' refers to the degree of congruence between the informants, in this case parents and professionals, and not to the accuracy of the information gathered, nor to the reliability between raters, rather to the confirmation of the fact that there is something to be learned from these profiles of agreement and disagreement between parents and professional, who observe the child from different perspectives. If it is important to obtain information from different resources, then the presence of congruence or the lack thereof between the different resources can be both informative and important (11). Therefore the present research examined disagreement as well as agreement between parents and professionals.

In those cases in which the parents and professionals disagreed with regard to language abilities, parents tended to overestimate their child's language skills. This finding supports Dinnebeil and Rule's (11) review, in which they found that when disagreement emerged between parents' and professionals' assessments, the parents' judgments tended to be higher than the professionals'. The suggested explanation was that the parents' judgments of their children's development based on broader contexts, in which the children's behavior can be seen more clearly than in the assessment context, which is a contrived and specific setting. An alternative explanation posits that parents' are less objective that professionals regarding their children, but since we were not assessing the accuracy of the reporting this point will not be addressed here. Voelker et al (17) reported a possible third explanation in her study of congruence in parent and teacher ratings of adaptive behavior in low functioning children. She found that parents were apt to assess a skill as present or absent and not as emerging. So it is possible that the parents observed a particular behavior only once but would report that it exists. Similarly, parents may report that a skill exists even if it is still developing, and may not be advanced enough to receive a passing score on a standardized assessment.

In contrast to previous findings that parents may lessen abnormality , in the present research in those cases in which the parents and the professionals disagreed regarding their assessment of diagnostic characteristics of autism, parents did not tend to describe their children as more or less autistic than the profile which emerged from the professionals' testing. That may be the result of the fact that parents of children with autism are often suspicious that there is something different in their child's development before the diagnosis is formally assigned (19) Such awareness may limit expectations from their child, and may result in realistic assessments of the children's autism symptoms which may be comparable to the professionals' assessments. Thus, in the present study, the parents did not tend to report autism diagnostic characteristics as less pathological than the professionals.

One of the more interesting results of the study was the difference which emerged in the cases in which the parents and professionals disagreed. When professionals diagnose a child, adolescent or adult with autism, they use the population of children with autism as the criterion group for comparison of diagnostic characteristics, whereas, parents compare children's characteristics to what they have learned and know from the general population. This difference can cause professionals to judge the children as less pathological compared to other children with autism as a group of reference, while the parents judge these same characteristics as more pathological compared to the general population as a group of reference. Thus, there was no tendency of parents to estimate their children in a less pathological way than the professionals behaviorally, while in assessing language skills both the parents and the professionals use typical development as their reference point.

The present research also attempted to investigate other correlates which may be associated with degrees of dis/agreement between parents and professionals. Previously, discrepancies between mothers and child perceptions have been found to be related to parenting and to predict child behavioral problems (29,30). First, child related variables were examined,and although chronological ages are less relevant than mental ages for research in atypical populations, including autism, it was decided to examine this variable in the present study. It was reasonable to assume that the degree of agreement between parents and professionals might be related to the subjects' chronological ages, although in the present research, the degree of agreement between parents and professionals regarding the diagnostic characteristics and the children's language skills was not related to the children's chronological age. This finding that the degree of agreement was not related to the children's chronological ages, might strengthen the claim that mental age is more significant and meaningful than the children's chronological age, when assessing skill levels. Unlike chronological age, mental age was found to significantly correlate with the degree of agreement between parents and professionals regarding the children's language skills. At the same time, there was no similar correlation regarding the children's diagnostic characteristics, which seem not to be age dependent. Regarding the children's language skills, it was found that as the children's mental ages increased, the degree of agreement between parents and professionals was higher. This finding may be explained by the fact that mental age reflects cognitive abilities one of which is language capabilities, which was assessed in the present study. Thus, when the children's language skills are higher, it is easier both for the parents and professionals to estimate them and to agree. On the other hand, as the children's language skills are lower, the professionals might assess them as low, but the parents might estimate their language skills as higher than they really are, because of the broader context and familiarity; they understand them better. Thus, degree of agreement between parents and professionals is low in the children with the lower mental ages.

The profile is quite different when analyzing informant differences regarding diagnostic characteristics, where no association between mental age and autism symptoms was revealed. Children's diagnostic characteristics may be more consistent over contexts, with more outstanding behavioral manifestation associated with autism. Therefore, it is possible that the short time and the limited context in which the professionals and children meet do not significantly influence the assessment of autistic symptomotology.

Parental variables were also examined in the present research and no correlations were found between experience in child rearing or knowledge of developmental milestones and the degree of agreement between parents and professionals regarding the children's diagnostic characteristics and language skills. It seems like the difference between degrees of agreement in assessing language skills and diagnostic behavioral characteristics represents a true difference in perspective, which parents and professionals bring to the assessment process.

Conclusion

In sum, the present research results support the basic perception that when parents and professionals estimate children with autism, they reach high degree of agreement, despite the fact that they have differing perspectives. Therefore, one might be tempted to assume that one source of information would be enough. But, although the degree of agreement is high, there is not complete agreement and the information from one source complements the information from the other. Thus, the findings support the need to integrate parental reporting in the assessment process as an additional source of information to the information gathered from clinical testing.

Each informant has a different but valid perspective regarding the behavior being assessed, and therefore it is important to maintain the contribution of each to the assessment process. In other words, a behavior will be considered as present when it is reported at least by one rater or informant(3). Bagnato and Neisworth (31) described the assessment process as information which is gathered from many resources and coined the term 'convergent assessment'. The purpose of this kind of assessment is to synthesize information gathered from multiple resources, and to produce the most valid assessment of the child's development and abilities.

Another way of dealing with information from different informants is to assume that each informant reports differently on specific behaviors, resulting in a complementary profile. It is also important to relate both to the type of behavior being assessed and to the context in which the behavior is expressed. Thus, it is important to systematically check those items for which there are discrepencies to disagreements and to reach a decision regarding each behavior or ability. In order to do so, it is important to take into consideration the context in which the assessment occurred the informant and manner in which the information was collected and therefore by perceiving the information as cogent and supplementary and not as having to see one as correct , the child may be understood more comprehensively.

Future research should focus on trying to identify those items with high and those items with low degrees of agreement between parents and professionals, across individuals and levels of function. By focusing on the content of such items, the profiles revealed in future research might help to identify common issues and areas of contents where there are high or low degrees of agreements between parents and professionals. Findings of this type could be seminal in building assessment processes which use information from multiple informants effectively and differentially.

Finally, the present research results emphasize the importance of parents' and professionals' collaborative work. In particular, in autism, which is characterized by social and communication impairments, it is important to get information from as many of the informants connected to the child and from all the situations in the child's life in order to reach the best diagnosis and assessment possible. In addition, because the disability begins to be identified at a young age, it is important to diagnose the children as early as possible in order to begin appropriate early intervention. A diagnosis that is a result of information from many sources might help the parents deal better with understanding the diagnosis. Also, the parents' active participation in the assessment process might ease the tension which often emerges after receiving the diagnosis. Thus, cooperation among parents and professionals in the diagnosis and assessment process of children with autism is extremely valuable for everyone – for the professionals, for the parents and most importantly, for the children.

References

[1] Lord C, McGee JP. Educating children with autism. Washington, DC: Natl. Acad. Press, 2001.

[2] Achenbach TM, McConaughy SH, Howell CT. Child/adolescent behavioral and emotional problems: Implications of cross-informant correlations for situational specificity. Psychol. Bull 1987;101:213-32.

[3] Hart EL, Lahey BB, Loeber R, Hanson KS. Criterion validity of informants in the diagnosis of disruptive behavior disorders in children: A preliminary study. J. Consult. Clin. Psychol. 1994;62(2):410-4.

[4] Frick PJ, Silverhorn P, Evans C. Assessment of childhood anxiety using structured interviews: Patterns of agreement among in formants and association with maternal anxiety. Psychol. Assess 1994;6:372-9.

[5] Szatmari P, Archer L, Fisman S, Streiner DL. Parent and teacher agreement of pervasive developmental disorders. J. Autism Dev. Disord. 1994;24(6):703-17.

[6] De Los Reyes A, Kazdin AE. Informant discrepancies in the assessment of childhood psychopathology: A critical review, theoretical framework and recommendations for further study. Psychol. Bull 2005;131(4):483-509.

[7] Choudhury MS, Pimental SS, Kendall PC. Childhood anxiety disorders: Parent-child (dis)agreement using a structured interview for the DSM-IV. J. Amr. Acad. Child Adolesc. Psychiatr. 2003;42:957-64.

[8] Grills AE, Ollendick, TH. Issues in parent-child agreement:The case of structured diagnostic interviews. Clin. Child Fam. Psychiatr. Rev. 2002;5(1):57-83.

[9] Sessa FM, Avenevoli S, Steinberg L, Morris AS. Correspondence among informants on parenting: Preschool children, mothers, and observers. J. Fam. Psychol. 2001;15:53-68.

[10] Dinnebeil LA, Rule S. Congruence between parents' and professionals' judgments about the development of young children with disabilities: A review of the literature. Topics Early Childhood Spec. Educ. 1994;14(1):1-25.

[11] Stone WL, Rosenblum JL. A comparison of teacher and parent view of autism. J. Autism Dev. Disord. 1988;18(3):403-14.

[12] Chamberlain P, Reid JB. Parent observation and report of child symptoms. Behav. Assess 1987;9:97-109.

[13] Stone WL, Lemanek KL. Parental report of social behaviors in autistic preschoolers. J. Autism Dev. Disord. 1990;20(4):513-22.

[14] Byrne JM, Backman JE, Smith IM. Developmental assessment: The clinical use and validity of parental report. J. Pediatr. Psychol. 1986;11(4):549-59.

[15] Stiles J. On the nature of informant judgments in inventory measures: And so what is it you want to know? Monogr. Soc. Res. Child Dev. 1994;59(5):180-4.

[16] Miller JF, Sedey AL, Miolo G. Validity of parent report measures of vocabulary development for children with Down syndrome. J. Speech Hearing Res. 1995;38:1037-44.

[17] Voelker SL, Shore DL, Lee CH, Szuszkiewicz TA. Congruence in parent and teacher ratings of adaptive behavior of low functioning children. J. Dev. Phys. Disabil. 2000;12(4):367-76.

[18] Krug DA, Arick J, Almond, P. Behavioral checklist for identifying severely handicapped individuals with high levels of autistic behavior. J. Child. Psychiatr. Psychol. 1980;21:221-9.

[19] Shulman C. Bridging the process between diagnosis and treatment. In: Gabriels R, Hill D, eds. Autism from research to individualized practice. London: Jessica Kingsley, 2002:25-46.

[20] American Psychiatric Association. Diagnostic and Statistical Manual of Mental Disorders, (DSM-IV), 4th ed. Washington DC.: Am. Psychiatr. Assoc., 1994.

[21] World Health Organization. The ICD classification of mental and behavioral disorders: Clinical descriptions and diagnostic guidelines (ICD-10). Geneva: World Health Organization, 1992.

[22] Lord C, Risi S, Lambrecht L, Cook E, Leventhal B, Dilavore P, Pickles A, Rutter M. The Autism Diagnostic Observation Schedule-Generic: A standard measure of social and communication deficits associated with the spectrum of autism. J. Autism Dev. Disord. 2000;30:205-23.

[23] Lord C, Rutter M, Le Couteur A. Autism Diagnostic Interview - Revised: A revised version of a diagnostic interview for caregivers of individuals with possible pervasive developmental disorders. J. Autism Dev. Disord. 1994;24(5): 659-85.

[24] Mullen E. Mullen Scales of Early Learning. Circle Pines, MN: Am. Guidance Serv., 1992.

[25] Sparrow S, Balla D, Cicchetti DV. Vineland Adaptive Behavior Scales. Circle Pines, MN: Am. Guidance Serv., 1984.

[26] Hedrick DL, Prather EM, Tobin AR. Sequenced inventory of communication development. Seattle, WA: Univ Wash Press, 1984.

[27] Humphreys LE, Ciminero AR. Parent report of child behavior: A review. J. Clin. Child Psychol. 1979;8(1):56-63.

[28] Angold A, Weissman M, John K, Merikangas KR, Prusoff, BA., et al. Parents and child reports of depressive symptoms in children in low and high risk for depression. J. Child Psychol. Psychiatr. 1987;28:901-15.

[29] Chi T, Hinshaw SP. Mother child relationships of children with ADHD. J. Abn. Child Psychol. 2002;30: 387-400.

[30] Ferdinand RF, van der Ende J, Verhaulst FC. Parent-adolescent disagreement regarding psychopatholgy in adolescents from the general population as a risk factor for adverse outcome. J. Abn. Psychol. 2004;113: 198-206.

[31] Bagnato, SJ, Neisworth, JT. Assessment for early intervention: Best practices for professionals. New York: Guilford, 1991.

In: Understanding Autism Spectrum Disorder
Editors: Ditza A Zachor and Joav Merrick

ISBN: 978-1-62081-353-9

Chapter 9

Joint construction of stories by high functioning children with autism: Using a technological setting

Judy Kupersmitt[1]*, Rachel Yifat[1], Eynat Gal[2], Nirit Bauminger[3], Oliviero Stock[4], Massimo Zancanaro[4], Fabio Pianesi[4] and Patrice L. (Tamar) Weiss[2]

[1]Department of Communication Sciences and Disorders, Faculty of Social Welfare and Health Sciences, University of Haifa, Mount Carmel, Haifa

[2]Department of Occupational Therapy, Faculty of Social Welfare and Health Sciences, University of Haifa, Mount Carmel, Haifa,

[3]School of Education, Bar Ilan University, Ramat Gan, Israel

[4]Fondazione Bruno Kessler – Instituto per la Ricerca Scientifica e Tecnologica, Italy

Abstract

This chapter examines the joint construction of stories across eight sessions, by three pairs of high-functioning children with ASD (autism spectrum disorder) using a unique technological setting designed to enhance collaboration. Stories are evaluated in terms of form and content. Preliminary findings show that stories increase in length by session, but they overall show poor local and global coherence, lacking either temporal or causal connections between subsequent propositions. They are also composed of few events and include a large proportion of repeated or reformulated clauses. More than half of the stories were enacted rather than narrated, as typical of dyadic storytelling. Analysis of the verbal interaction that leads to story construction shows that children did not plan or negotiate story construction. In turn, the adult intervention and support was required to

* Correspondence: Judy Kupersmitt, Department of Communication Sciences and Disorders, Faculty of Social Welfare and Health Sciences, University of Haifa, Mount Carmel, IL-31905 Haifa, Israel. Tel: 972 (0)4 8240111; E-mail address: judykup@bezeqint.net

continue with the story under certain circumstances. Findings are discussed in light of the contextual conditions and goals determined by the particular technological setting.

Introduction

The ability to participate in narrative activities is central to human nature and is critical to the development of communicative competence. When children engage in storytelling, they are bringing together thought, action, and feeling into an organized verbal framework (1,2). Forming part of more general socialization processes, narrative abilities emerge as embedded in conversation with significant others, and become one of the pillars of the child's general pragmatic development (3). Through storytelling, children learn to share experiences with others and recognize different perspectives of the same events; they begin to understand others' attitudes, emotions, knowledge and motivations (4). Moreover, narrative is a vehicle for the acquisition and development of particular ways to talk about events beyond the sentence level, first, in a conversational context with rich supportive input from an adult or peer partner (3), and later, as an autonomous text produced by children with little verbal support (5,6).

The analysis of narrative practices, therefore, represents a rich source for investigating the interactions between pragmatic, linguistic, and socio-cognitive abilities. This is particularly interesting with special populations, since these abilities may be affected, and interactions are less likely to occur. In children with autistic spectrum disorders (ASD), the target population of the current study, narrative abilities seem impaired relative to typically developing populations. Most of the narrative research in ASD has focused on basic narrative measures such as story length, structure, and use of cohesive devices, using direct elicitation methods such as retelling a puppet show or video sketch (7), a story from a wordless picture book (8,9) or telling narratives of personal experiences (10). When matched for language abilities with typically developing children or with children with developmental disabilities, no major differences were found in narrative length or sentence complexity. However, several studies have reported difficulties referencing mental states (11,12), expressing causal connections and using causal language to integrate narrative events into a thematically organized and elaborated whole (10,13). These last findings have been attributed to theory of mind deficits in children with autism, which may be related to their incapacity to both understand the listeners' needs and the underlying intentions, emotions and motivations of the characters in the narrative.

Eliciting narratives from children with autism is a difficult enterprise since these children lack a basic motivation to communicate with others, even when they have acquired some linguistic competence. They may also not experience the same pleasure as other children in experimental tasks designed to tap linguistic and particularly narrative knowledge. Therefore, gathering narrative data from children with autism needs to be tailored to the particular characteristics of this population. During the last decades there have been an increasing number of studies using computers for enhancing communication in autistic children (14,15).

These studies reported the benefit of computer aided learning on a range of socio-cognitive and language related behaviors, including improved attention, social interaction and motivation. Moreover, children with autism respond well to fixed visual cues and written words, making computerized environments an ideal arena for practicing language and communication skills. Motivated by research that used technological aids for storytelling with typical populations (16,17), a number of recent studies have designed software systems for children with autism in the context of narrative and social understanding (18-20). However, these studies are scarce and mostly assess individual narrative comprehension, aiming to identify different aspects of narrative that could be improved by intervention through interactive computer.

The present chapter reports on findings of a pilot investigation that examined the joint production of stories by three pairs of high-functioning children with ASD across eight sessions, using a unique computerized interface designed to enhance collaboration. Co-operative storytelling among typically developing children was examined particularly in educational contexts, where children were asked to generate common stories about different curriculum related topics (21).

Lately, a few studies have suggested that dyadic storytelling may have a variety of consequences, some of them beneficial (e.g., children have more fun, tell longer stories), and some of them negative (e.g., less cohesive stories, multiple character introduction) (22). In autism, co-operative storytelling is an innovative and potentially rich area of study, providing material on social interaction and understanding, language, role taking and pretence, as well as on narrative construction per se. The present chapter focuses on the effects of the computerized software on narrative co-production across sessions. Specifically, the narratives produced are evaluated according to central features of fictional narratives in terms of form and content. In addition, the study examines whether the children planned the stories while interacting around the StoryTable, as part of the dyadic task, and to what extent they were capable to create the narratives autonomously or they needed the adult's scaffolding and support. Addressing these questions may contribute to our understanding of the impact of computerized tools for further research, diagnosis and treatment of communication abilities in children with ASD, with an emphasis on the production of extended discourse.

Our study

Six Hebrew speaking boys with high functioning ASD, aged 9 to 11 participated in the study. The children were diagnosed according to the Diagnostic and Statistical Manual of Mental Disorders (fourth edition, APA 2000), further confirmed by the Childhood Autism Rating Scale (CARS) (23) or the Autism Diagnostic Interview-Revised (ADI-R) (24) which were administered to the parents of the children. Receptive vocabulary scores, using the Peabody Picture Vocabulary Test (PPVT), indicated performance about average. All the children were able to use language at least at the level of simple sentence construction and performed at Grade 2 levels in reading and writing tasks. Diagnosis was performed by a licensed psychologist and a speech therapist. The children attended a special education program within a typical elementary school, had experienced peer interactions with typically developing children as well as with other children with ASD, and were judged by educators as being socially competent. They all showed basic pragmatic skills and were able to engage in social interactions that require turn-taking, listening to each other and relating to the others' talk. None of them had physical disabilities or was receiving other types of social interventions in school at the time of the study.

Materials

The activity was performed using the StoryTable deployed through the Mistubishi Electronic Research Laboratory (MERL) DiamondTouch (DT) Table, a multi-user touchable interface that detects multiple simultaneous touches by two to four users (25, 26). The Story Table interface has been designed according to the symbol of ladybugs wandering around the table surface, differing in size and color according with their functions. One ladybug carries the backgrounds that will serve as the story setting (e.g., a forest, a castle, or a farm) and another ladybug carries the characters and objects that can be dragged onto the current background. A third type of ladybug of a different size and shape contains the audio snippets that will form the story. The audio snippets are dragged into the recorder and recorded independently by each child. An audio ladybug is "owned" by the child who recorded it. Yet, the two children may agree to release ownership of a ladybug by a multiple-user drag-and-drop action. The resulting story is the sequence of the audio snippets recorded in the ladybugs placed in the sequence of holes at the bottom edge of the interface. While each audio ladybug may be listened to individually, the story as a connected sequence of snippets can be listened to only if both the children touch the first ladybug in the sequence.

The StoryTable setting requires that participants agree on relevant steps to be taken during story construction (release the ownership of an audio ladybug, choose the background setting, or listen to the whole story) and make this physically explicit by joint actions. Thus, the very nature of the task requires children with ASD to engage in a number of social and verbal behaviors they most often refrain from.

Procedure

In order to operate the StoryTable, an 11-item skills checklist was developed and presented to the children prior to their selection for the study (27).

The skill rubric included such activities as selecting a background graphic, selecting and placing story characters, and recording segments of a story in one's own voice. Skill level thresholds for each task and general threshold score were established. Only children who achieved scores beyond the threshold were included in the study.

Before the sessions started, children focused first on learning to operate the StoryTable using a written list of StoryTable functions and rules. All of the children learned to successfully operate the StoryTable after this short training. They were then divided into three pairs as suggested by their teacher, based on social preferences and competence.

The activity around the StoryTable was performed during eight sessions over a period of three weeks. Following the requirements of the collaborative task, children selected together the background for the story they wanted to narrate, and then composed it while taking turns, recording the narrative output via the StoryTable audio snippets.

Sessions ended after each child narrated for three alternating turns. The adult guiding the interaction actively supported the children with the technical management of the interface and provided verbal reinforcements when needed. Contributions of the adult to story construction were meant to be reduced to a minimum.

All sessions were videotaped using a digital video camera. Language samples were transcribed verbatim to a data sheet, specifying the turns taken by each child, and included the conversation around the story and the story itself.

Coding categories

The co-constructed stories were evaluated according to a set of categories adapted from different studies aimed at understanding storytelling competence in a wide range of typical and atypical populations in various settings (5,2).

These categories are meant to assess the typicality and overall quality of stories, along the dimensions detailed below.

- *Story length*: measured in number of clauses, where a clause refers to 'any unit that contains a unified predicate that expresses a single situation (activity, event, state)' (5, p. 660). Proportions for all narrative measures were calculated out of total clauses in order to control for the influence of story length.
- *Clause linkage*: the ordering of the information in sequences that are temporally or thematically coherent. Temporal coherence means that two events are arranged in a certain temporal order (e.g., 'the king went on a walk and he found snails'). Thematic coherence divides into informational -- were situations have some kind of thematically connection (e.g., 'She's getting ready for school. She's doing her homework') and causal -- were propositions are linked conceptually or explicitly by causal connectors (e.g., 'Mogli was sad because the monkeys kidnapped him'). Linkage was evaluated across clauses in subsequent turns to examine whether propositions were relevant to the preceding ones. Causal relations were considered global if they related to an explicit goal or problem (28). Within this category, we coded use of conjunctions (e.g., and, but, then, because) (29,30) and of referential markers to introduce characters and maintain the reference to them across clauses and turns (29).
- *Information status*: the amount of novel versus non-novel information, including repetitions and reformulations.
- *Tense of clauses*: marked as past (e.g., jumped), present (e.g., jumps), future (will jump) or other (to jump, have to jump, would jump). Use of past tense defines stories as a specific genre distinct from descriptions (which require use of present tense) or conversations about the immediate context, where tense may alternate between present, past, and future.
- *Enacted versus 3rd person stories*: pretend play stories (where narrators enact the characters' role) versus prototypical storytelling (where the narrator is distinct from the protagonist/s).
- *Story content*: the type of information conveyed in each clause (31,32) including introductions (e.g., 'I'm going to tell a story about a princess'); events (e.g., 'Mogli met the elephant'); descriptions (e.g., 'the princess and the knight, they had a really wonderful wedding'); and internal states (e.g., 'it was not nice to him').

In order to look for evidence of story planning and adult scaffolding, meta-narrative utterances within the conversation around the story table were analyzed. These were identified as specific talk around some aspect related to story construction, including story structure, content, characters, or language, as well as evaluative comments on the story (31). All transcriptions were coded independently by the authors and by four final year undergraduate students in the Dept. of Communication Disorders for each of the categories, reaching an inter-rater agreement of above 90%.

Our findings

This section starts with presenting results on the effects of the interface on the quality of the stories produced (section 3.1) and follows with the results on story planning and adult scaffolding (section 3.2).

Evaluation of stories

Results for story length and clause linkage are presented for each of the sessions to examine for possible effects of task experience. For the rest of the categories, stories are considered all together across sessions, while referring to specific sessions for the purposes of illustrations and qualitative descriptions. For all the results, quantitative findings are interspersed with illustrative examples and interpretations. Figure 1 shows a homogeneous behavior among the three pairs during the first session (about 10 clauses), with an inconsistent increase in narrative length from session 2 onward. Pair 2 told the longest stories, ranging from 10 clauses during the first session to 50 clauses during session 7.

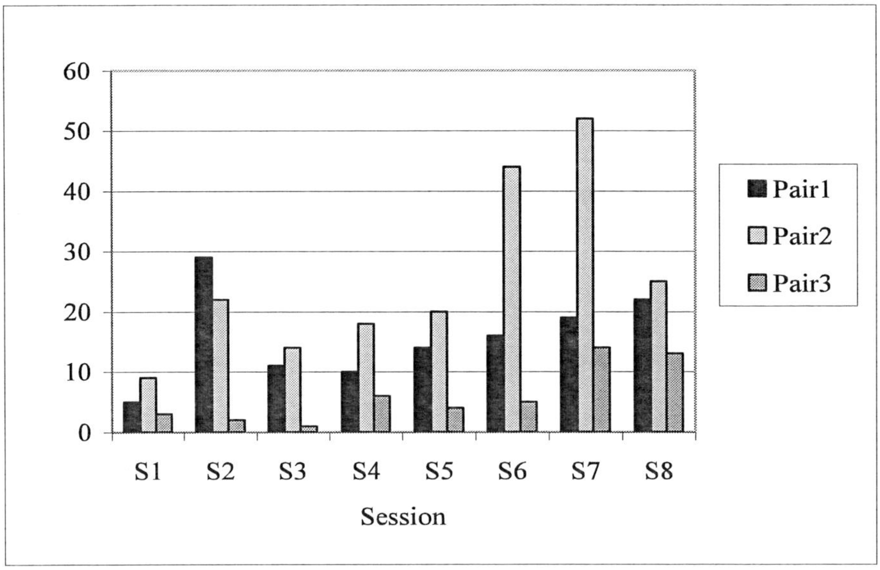

Figure 1: Total number of clauses, by session and pair.

Pair 1 showed a sharp increase in session 2 (30 clauses) but remained steady for the next sessions with a mean of 15 clauses. Pair 3 narrated the shortest stories reaching only 10 clauses during their last session.

This likely indicates individual differences in dealing with the narrative task, which are particularly noticeable once the children became familiar with the novel technical setting. Although story length is not necessarily indicative of the quality of stories (see sections below), it may reflect the children's increased attention to the goal of the activity.

Clause linkage was examined to reveal the ability of the children to produce thematically linked segments in story production, while relating to the information provided by their partner. Results on clause linkage are shown in figure 2.

Figure 2 shows the low proportions of linked clauses, where pairs 1 and 2 made the highest proportions (38% and 47% across sessions out of total clauses, respectively) and pair 3 made only 8%. Clauses were less connected in the first session (28%, 11% and 0% of clauses for pairs 1, 2 and 3, respectively), with no clear improvement across sessions. Pair 2, for example, reached as high as 82% of linked clauses during session 3 but then decreased to only 29% during session 6 and up to 63% during session 7.

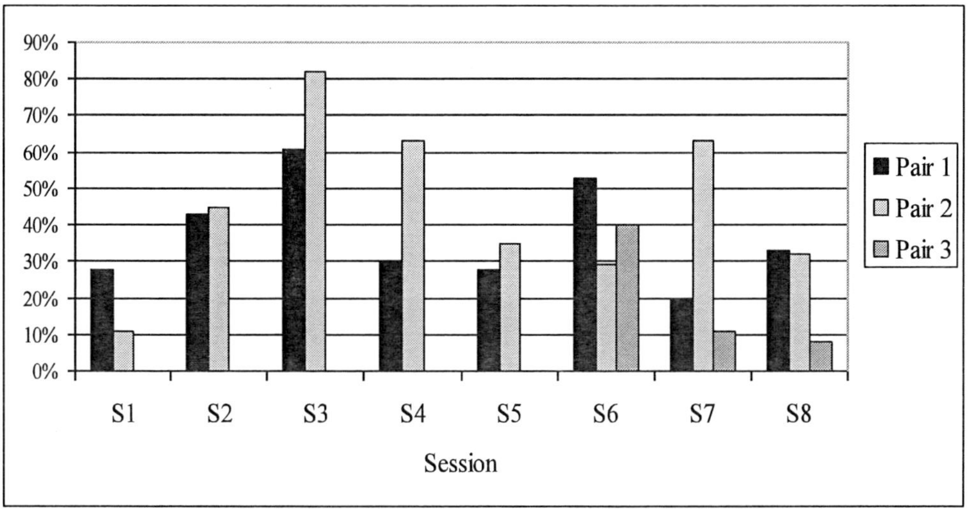

Figure 2: Percentage of linked clauses, by session and pair.

Clause linkage in the most connected story is illustrated in example 1 below. Throughout the examples, letters in the first column stand for the names of the participants. In the second column, N stands for narrative clauses (i.e. the clauses in the co-constructed story) and C stands for conversation. Adult contributions are explicitly stated. A free translation of the texts is shown in the third column, following the original Hebrew text only where relevant.

The clauses in example 1 are linked temporally (underlined items show use of temporal conjunctions) or thematically by an enabling relation (N7= the tiger drowns; N8= the sharks devour the tiger). A closer look at the proportion of clause linkage between turns and within turns for pairs 1 and 2 revealed that clause linkage occurred mostly within turns (around 80%), that is, between clauses mentioned by the same child. This means that children were telling independent stories rather than collaborating (as further illustrated in example 2 by pair 1).

Example 1: Clause linkage, pair 2 ("E" and "O"), session 3

E	N1	'Once *Kofiko* (a monkey) went to the sea
	N2	and after *it* went to the sea
	N3	and swam there
	N4	*it* saw *Shirhan* the terrible tiger
O	N5	This *Kofiko* zaps *Shirhan* on *its* tail
	N6	and then *it* went to the water…to the sea
	N7	and *it* drowned
E	C1	Yes, but you forgot to make frightening noises
Adult		Elad goes on.
E	N8	The sharks devoured *the tiger*
O	N9	*Mogli* climbed the tree
	N10	and *Kofiko* saw *Morli*
E	C2	Not *Morli*, Mogli
	N9	mm…*Kofiko* said to *Mogli*
	N10	Hello, said *Mogli* to *Kofiko*
O	N11	A bear came
	N12	*Mogli*! *Kofiko*! "What are you doing there in the jungle?"

In the excerpt below, it is clear that child "R" shifted the topic of the story told by child "Y", as shown by the introductive clause N5 'I'll tell a story' and the new characters introduced in N6 (marked in bold). Child "Y" continued with his own story in the subsequent turn starting with N10, by reformulating clauses N3 and N4, thus creating two parallel stories. Within turns, clauses show some level of thematic or temporal linking, though choice of wrong conjunctions and ambiguous use of pronouns make the thematic relations less clear.

Example 2: Clause linkage within turns, pair 1 ("Y" and "R"), session 2

Y	N1	The king went on a walk
	N2	and he found snails
	N3	and he enjoyed the walk
	N4	and he had fun (3 clauses by Y with repeated content skipped)
R	N5	I'll tell a story
	N6	**Two knights** fight with **ten dragons**
	N7	but they didn't give up
	N8	but they managed to keep away from them
	N9	and then they killed them
Y	N10	The king was happy with his walk
	N11	and he enjoyed

Results on use of different conjunctions revealed that 'and' was preferred among the three pairs, but was used in no more than 12% of total narrative clauses in Pair 1 and much less in pairs 2 and 3. Other conjunctions such as 'then', 'so/then', or 'because', were used in less than 5% of total clauses in all pairs. Around one third of the conjunctions used did not reflect a clear temporal or thematic connection between the adjacent clauses.

Clause linkage was further evaluated by use of referential expressions for character presentation and maintenance. Reference was analyzed for pair 1 only, since they had the highest proportion of narratives told in 3rd person perspective (as further detailed below). Results showed that 66% of total referential expressions served to maintain the reference between successive clauses, both within turns and across consecutive turns (assigned to each child alternatively for recording the narrative, as specified in section 2.3 above). Out of this total, half (33%) served to maintain the reference to characters within turns. Across turns, as expected, children used full noun phrases, as they generally resumed the story after managing with technical or organizational procedures related to the activity. The remaining half was divided into (1) use of full nouns for character re-introduction after another character was referred to in the anterior turn (see example 2 above), as well as for adding new characters, and (2) pronouns deployed ambiguously across turns (see example 2, clauses 7-9).

Interestingly, the ability to maintain the reference to characters is not positively correlated with the ability to link the clauses thematically (correlation coefficient = 0.189). For example, during sessions 5 and 7, children managed to maintain the reference in more than 80% of the cases, but the stories produced during these sessions were poorly connected in thematic terms (with only 20-30% of linked clauses, as shown in figure 2). Moreover, many instances of reference maintenance occurred in repeated or reformulated clauses, as further illustrated below.

Thus, one may only tentatively suggest that the ability to maintain the reference to characters is less damaged than the ability to coherently relate information encoded in subsequent clauses. Probably, the fact that the children set up the characters before they started to tell the stories, avoided introduction of multiple characters and facilitated reference maintenance.

In summary, results on clause linkage showed mainly informational links and referential chains at a local level, but less so at a global level, as further discussed below.

The coding of information status revealed that about 20-40% of total clauses among all pairs were repeated or reformulated, either as requested by the adult when recording was not activated, or self-initiated by the children. Pair 3 showed the highest proportion of verbatim repeated clauses (27% compared to 7-8% for pairs 1 and 2), a further corroboration of their less coherent narratives, as shown in figure 2. Their stories were not only shorter but also composed mainly of repeated clauses. For example, the story produced during session 1 consisted of a single clause -- 'one day (I) went to mom's grocery' -- repeated seven times with slight changes (e.g., 'one day I went to the grocery with mom/dad').

The story narrated during session 4 included the clause 'the king died' repeated five times out of total of 7 clauses. On the other hand, reformulated clauses such as those including some kind of content or language change should not be treated as mere stereotyped linguistic behavior, as illustrated in example 3 below. This example from an enacted story shows that N1 was repeated by the second child "O" in the subsequent clauses, as requested by his partner in C1. While these repetitions suspended story elaboration, they may reflect instances of collaboration in the joint production of the story, and, not less important, awareness of the verbal productions, of their meaning and contribution to the collaborative storytelling activity.

Thus, this excerpt shows that when one of the speakers changes a linguistic form (e.g., the preposition 'like' for the preposition 'with') his partner corrects him according to the model provided before.

Example 3: Repeated and reformulated clauses initiated by the children, pair 2 ("E" and "O"), session 7

E	N1	*Uf! anaxnu ovdim kmo xamorim* 'Oof! we are working like donkeys'
	N2	*yala! Al tagidu she atem xamorim* 'come on! Don't say you're donkeys' (10 narrative clauses skipped)
E	C1	*tagid anaxnu ovdim mamash kmo xamorim* 'say: we are working really like donkeys'
O	N3	*anaxnu ovdim mamash im xamorim* 'we are working really with donkeys'
	N4	*anaxnu ovdim mamash im xamorim* 'we are working really with donkeys'
E	C2	*lo mamash im xamorim, mamash kmo xamorim!* 'not really with donkeys, really like donkeys'!
O	N5	*i efshar, anaxnu ovdim kmo xamorim* 'We can't, we work like donkeys'

Reformulations served also as a discourse strategy to uptake the flow of the story from turn to turn, as illustrated in example 4 from pair 1.

Example 4: Repeated and reformulated clauses initiated by the children, pair 1 ("Y" and "R"), session 7

Y	N1	*Yom exad ha-kof* (=kofim)...*xatfu et Mogli* 'one day the monk...(=monkeys) kidnapped Mogli'
	N2	*ve ze lo haya lo nayim* 'and (it) was not nice to him'
		(12 turns skipped where children and adult deal with technicalities)
R	N3	*hayu harbe kofim* '(there) were a lot of monkeys'
	N4	*xatfu et Mogli* '(they) kidnapped Mogli'
	N5	*ve asu...ve asu harbe hishtolelut* 'and (they) went...(they) went pretty wild '
	N6	*ve haya lo nayim le-Mogli* 'and (it) was not nice to Mogli'

Example 4 shows that child "R" reformulated and even expanded the story started by child "Y" in N1 and N2. Therefore, reformulations may be reflecting creative linguistic and discourse strategies adopted by the children in the online production of stories. These gave children a platform for story elaboration, change in agency perspective and tense of verb (e.g., 'the dragon fought with the knight' versus 'two knights fight with ten dragons' in example 2), and use of different lexical items or connectors.

In order to distinguish storytelling from enacted stories, the proportion of 3rd person versus enacted stories was calculated out of the total number of clauses. Pair 1 told 3rd person stories exclusively, pair 2 engaged mostly in enactment (76%), and pair 3 showed mixed types, where no dominant perspective was chosen. The high proportion of enacted stories may be due to the interactive task, where role-taking is more common than in individual storytelling.

Also, choice of story perspective seems related to the different story backgrounds. Backgrounds such as jungles and castles brought about 3rd person stories, while more realistic backgrounds such as a house with people sitting in it or a school setting resulted in enacted stories. Individual differences in storytelling abilities and preferences were noted when pairs of children who chose the same background engaged in different telling modes. For example, a castle background with a princess, a knight and dragons served as a basis for

3rd person stories in pair 1, for enactment in pair 2, and for repetition of one single proposition in pair 3.

Story perspective entailed particular tense choices. Use of past tense was favored in 3rd person narratives, confirming the claim that past tense is indeed a key feature of temporal reference in storytelling (5,33).

Present and other tenses, however, were used when children engaged in enactment rather than in storytelling. Starting with pair 1, six of their stories were based on a background depicting either a jungle (from the Jungle Book) or a castle with typical characters. The stories based on these two backgrounds were told in the past tense entirely. Interestingly, when producing a story based on a more realistic scenario, this same pair opened the story in the past but continued in the present tense, as illustrated in example 5.

Other uses of the present in this same pair occurred when referring to actions that implied a certain duration or indicated a process (eat, climb, play), as opposed to those that encoded non-durative events (found, took). In this case, past and present tenses were used alternatively, reflecting picture description rather than storytelling, as reported in previous studies about choice of dominant tense in narratives produced by preschool children (5)

Example 5: Shift from past to present tense, pair 1 ("R" and "Y"), session 4

R	N1	'Once there were many children at school
R	N2	the children in school love date cake
Y	N3	soon the children eat (=are going to eat) breakfast
R	N3	the children wake up'

Pair 2 used the present tense in 61% of the clauses since their stories were enacted in seven out of the eight sessions. The only 3rd person story they produced was told in the past tense and was based on the jungle background. Other tenses used included the future tense (e.g., 'what do you want? That I will-be (=me to be) bored all day at school?'); and infinitives (e.g., '(we) want summer holidays, without doing problems'). For pair 3, a mixed pattern was observed, with shifts from past to present tense where children described habitual activities rather than engaging in storytelling. Finally, stories were analyzed in terms of their content to examine what children talked about. Results show that overall, stories were poor in events. Pair 1 reached a mean of only 38% of clauses encoding an event, and pairs 2 and 3 even less (33% and 26%, respectively). Taking all 3rd person stories, calculations of the mean proportion of content types revealed that these were composed of different types including introductions (22%), reference to internal states and descriptions (28%), and events (32%) , as illustrated by example 6, by pair 1.

Example 6 shows that children seemed to grasp the conventions of storytelling, as seen by their consistent use of narrative introductions (e.g., child "R" in N1, N6 and N11).

However, these introductions did not serve to set up the scene for plot development but rather launched one or two isolated events (e.g., 'Mogli walked and found the tiger'), alternating with reference to behavioral states of characters (e.g., 'it had fun'). The analyses of the transcripts revealed neither mention of the motivations of the actions performed by the characters, nor mention of conflicts to be solved or goals to be achieved, what resulted in locally rather than globally connected stories. An interesting finding was the high proportion of clauses encoding other types of content such as mention of future events (e.g., 'I'm gonna go and burn you up'), questions (e.g., 'what? Do you mean to shoot me arrows?'), and commands (e.g., 'go on working immediately!'), reaching as high as 36% of total narrative clauses, including enacted stories.

Example 6: Story content, pair 1 ("R" and "N"), session 3

R	N1	One time Mogli walked (=was walking)
	N2	(he) found the tiger
	N3	devoured him
R	C1	On the tree (pointing to screen)
Y	N4	Out of the trees came a snake and...
R	C2	This is Balu (pointing)
Y	N5	And (it) helped Mogli
R	N6	One time Balu and Mogli took three...a lot of monkeys
	N7	kidnapped them
Adult		Mogli disappeared (from screen). Pick someone else.
R	C3	Balu (picks character)
Y	N8	The elephant roared
	N9	and enjoyed
	N10	and it had fun
R	C4	Monkeys (picks character)
R	N11	One time the monkeys kidnapped Mogli
Y	N12	Balu climbed the tree close to Mogli
	N13	and was angry at the monkeys

The low level of event clauses together with low levels of temporal and causal sequences resulted in stories lacking a plot, even those created out of shared scripts (such as the Jungle Book). Most of the clauses reflected that although the children had internalized some narrative conventions and the roles of the characters depicted in the story (e.g., that monkeys kidnapped Mogli and that knights fought with monsters), they were not able to elaborate these actions into more complex episodes. This differs from what has been reported by other studies on the ability of children to create globally coherent stories (34) or embellish and elaborate them (35) in the course of dyadic or group scripted storytelling.

Story planning and adult's involvement with the task

Counting meta-narrative comments by the children revealed little involvement in planning the story as part of the collaborative task. Pair 2 ("E" and "O") was the most collaborative in the conversation around the story (a total of 28 comments across sessions), increasing with task experience (from 2 comments in sessions 1-4 to a mean of 10 in sessions 5-8). Interestingly, this pair engaged mostly in enactment, and so their comments resemble the negotiation during pretend play, where children suggest to one another what to say, as illustrated in example 7.

This example shows that child "E" guided child "O" through story production, and that he was attentive to his partner's responses. This is more typical of pretend play were coherence is achieved by means of a dialogic negotiation in the character's voice – here between the children and the woman chosen as characters (35).

Example 7: Negotiation around the story, pair 2 ("E" and "O"), session 7

E	You will be the children that say: "oof! We work like donkeys all the time", say: "we work like donkeys all the time"	
O	N1	You are donkey-like children!
	N2	Not true, you're a donkey-like woman!
	N3	Not true, you are donkeys!
E	Say: "we work like donkeys"	
O	N5	Work like donkeys that you are!
E	No, "we work like donkeys"	

A small number of comments were related to the language, as shown previously in example 1 (e.g.,'not Morli, Mogli') and in example 3 (e.g., 'not really with donkeys, really like donkeys'!), all produced by the same pair. These few comments may reflect instances of collaboration and joint attention, where at least one of the children in the pair is carefully attentive to the partner's contribution in the process of story co-production. Pairs 1 and 3 showed no instances of story planning, except for one single session by pair 1 were one child suggests the topic of the story (e.g. "tell a story about a king").

Findings on adult's meta-narrative comments show that the adult got involved in story construction – though this involvement was meant to be minimized – to enhance continuation of the story. Scaffolding seems not to be prompted by chance but related to certain patterns of storytelling and to overall conversational abilities of the children. For example, 3rd person narratives (which occurred mostly in pair 1, as detailed in the above section) demanded more scaffolding than enacted narratives, as shown in the following example.

Example 8: Adult scaffolding, pair 1 ("R" and "Y"), session 6

R	N1	One wolf found a little baby
Adult	C1	Is that all? What did it do with the baby? A wolf found a little baby and what?
R	N2	It took him to a cave
Adult	C2	It took him to a cave. Did it call him Mogli?
11 turns skipped related to the management with the task		
Adult	C3	(*Turns to the other child "Y" who gets the turn*) Do you remember what it did? Where did it take him to?
Y	N3	It took him to the jungle
	N4	and Mogli ate bananas
6 turns skipped related to the management with the task		
Adult	C4	(*Turns again* to "R") We told that the baby was in the cave and "Y" told that Mogli ate bananas, right? So what do you want to tell now?
R	N5	He's playing with Balu the bear in the jungle
Adult	C5	He's playing with Balu the bear in the jungle. And what else?
R	N6	He's playing with Balu
	N7	and then he eats a lot of bananas with Balu

Example 8 shows that the adult encourages children to continue with the story. Two main strategies of scaffold are identified: a) asking for more information (e.g., "what else?" or "what did he do after that?"); and b) resuming with the flow of the story when shifting turns, especially after long interruptions due to the management with the task. In this last case the adult usually reminds the children about the content of the previous narrative clauses. Example 9 shows a different effect of the adult's involvement, this time during an enacted story.

In this example, the adult orients the child towards leaving enactment and engaging in more traditional storytelling, as evident in the question "what happened after…?" However, the children do not seem attentive to this guidance and continue each of them with his own strategy, where "O" repeats what his partner said before and "E" continues with the enacted dialogue between the characters. Finally, notwithstanding the attempts of the adult to enhance the story to continue, the children failed to respond to this initiative, as illustrated in example 10, typical of most of the interactions by pair 3.

Example 9: Adult scaffolding, pair 2 ("E" and "O"), session 4

E	N1	"Excuse me lady, don't you think you have to do a little homework?
	N2	What are you standing there all day?
	N3	Don't be so lazy
	N4	Go and do your homework, and that's it"
Adult	C1	(*Turns to the other child "O"*) What happened after the neighbors said this to the girl? What did the girl say?
O	N5	*Her neighbors told the girl (c.f. the neighbors told the girl) "go and do your homework and that's it"
Adult	C2	(*Turns again to "E"*) And what about the neighbors? What did they do?
E	N6	"I'm all day doing homework and homework and homework.
	N7	What do you want?
	N8	I'm all day doing homework
	N9	I'm going to burn you up"

Example 10: Adult scaffolding, pair 3 ("A" and "Ra"), session 4

Adult	C1	Come on, start telling the story about the enchanted spring
Ra	N1	An enchanted spring
Adult	C2	(*Turning to the other child "A" who is making noises on the microphone*) "You have to talk about the enchanted spring, sweetheart. What happened in the enchanted spring?"
A	N2	Dead king, dead king
Adult	C3	(*Turning to Ra*) "Can you think what happened in the spring?"
Ra	N3	One day he put into the spring three drops, four drops
Adult	C4	Good, very nice. (*Turning to A*) Now, do you remember how the story continued?
A	N4	Dead king.
7 turns skipped related to the management with the task		
Adult	C5	What do you what to tell about the magic drops
5 turns skipped related to the management with the task		
A	N5	Dead king.

Discussion

This pilot study explored the effect of a unique technological setting programmed to enhance peer collaboration on the co-construction of stories by high functioning children with ASD. This is particularly motivating since little is known about how children with ASD actually respond to each other in the joint construction of stories. The study focused on the evaluation of the narratives as products of the interaction around the setting. In addition, the study looked for evidence of story planning and adult involvement during the interaction leading to the construction of stories. The results presented here are preliminary, and as such, the interpretation of findings is limited by the exploratory nature of the study.

The findings on narrative abilities as reflected in the narrative produced are consistent with those reported in previous studies. For 3rd person stories, the findings revealed almost no thematic progress, with poor temporal and causal connection of propositions, scarcely marked by overt connectivity markers. This was also reported in earlier studies on use of cohesive devices for organizing and connecting information in narratives produced by children with ASD (36, 37, 38). Moreover, stories were characterized by the use of inappropriate, 'bizarre', and disconnected utterances, abundant repetitions, and lack of elaboration, which may reflect underlying pragmatic difficulties (7,12). However, when comparing results, one should be aware of the considerable differences in elicitation procedures. The setting proposed here demanded collaborative story construction while being attentive to the set of pre-defined rules of the task, such as performing joint actions, taking turns, and agreeing on relevant steps. This is very different from the structured settings which characterized the studies above, with monologic narratives as products. Within this complex interactive setting, most children seemed aware of the pragmatic requirements involved in storytelling and of the transition from the conversation to the narrative, as reflected in their narrative introductions and the use of genre-related markers such as past tense and relatively appropriate referential strategies. On the other hand, most of the children seemed to be telling relatively independent -- rather than co-constructed -- stories. This is consistent with other studies on dyadic versus individual storytelling among preschoolers (22). In this context, it can also be explained in terms of the inability of children with ASD to relate to their partner's talk or be attentive to it. The large proportion of enacted stories seems also related to the dyadic condition, as found in studies where pairs or groups of children tended to enact the different roles in a fantasy situation rather than narrating it (17,39). Storytelling abilities seemed also affected by the different available backgrounds which served as visual prompts. These backgrounds may have tapped different narrative abilities and thus rendered different products (33). Backgrounds associated with shared scripts such as children's stories or films served as better storytelling prompts than others, as claimed by Sawyer (2002): "the skillful introduction of scaffolds – loose outlines of plots, or a shared memory of a fairy tale or movie – can help to guide children's natural collaborative improvisations into a narrative structure with global coherence" (p.343).

The StoryTable setting was meant to yield spontaneous, non-directed interaction, yet guided by a pre-defined set of functions and rules. This helped the children to be attentive to the dynamics of the interaction and turn-taking, and framed story construction. Pre-defined turns were represented by the recording ladybugs, and so became the most meaningful unit for the sequential arrangement of the child's contribution. However, this may have affected the conceptualization, motivation and ability of the children to develop a plot, since here, as opposed to other conversational contexts, turns were fixed and demanded continuous talk by each of the participants.

Storytelling ability presupposes knowledge of the basic structures that compose stories, a beginning, middle, and end, organized around a basic plot which generally includes a problem and a resolution. The mere collection of sentences strung together is not enough to create a good story. The analysis performed here revealed no evidence for story planning or negotiation of story aspects between turns. In this sense, children revealed no evidence of grasping the essential nature of stories, as an entity that has to be constructed according to particular characteristics. The reason for this seems yet unclear and requires further consideration. It is possible that, beyond the pragmatic deficit causing this poor understanding of the story as a whole composed of related sub-parts, the nature of the task may have posed a difficulty for the children to discuss any aspect of the story before recording the ladybug.

Related to this finding is the support provided by the adult and the conditions under which this support was evident. Data analysis showed that adult involvement was favored in 3rd person stories. Probably, on identifying a potential sequence of events, the adult would demand for more information to build a narrative. In addition, due to the relatively long interruptions between turns, it may be the case that the adult helped children resume the story line. These findings call attention to two significant domains that need further investigation: first, the reciprocal relationship between the child's performance and the adult's reactions, and second, from Vygotsky's perspective, the role of the adult's mediation and scaffolding strategies in facilitating the children's process of learning. Thus, even when the adult intervention was meant to be reduced to the minimum, tit seems that several factors within child-child interaction called for the adult's support.

Finally, the study suggests that storytelling is multi-faceted. There are many ways to tell stories, and each way requires different linguistic, cognitive, and pragmatic skills. In order to enhance storytelling in children with ASD as part of their communicative and social development, further research aimed at the developing intervention tools for engaging in storytelling experiences must be done. Technology offers a wide range of interactive options for these purposes. When working with typically developing children, the advantage of technological environments that demand collaboration lies in exposing peers to exchanging ideas and meaning negotiation. Such interaction requires attentiveness, empathy, and responsiveness to one's partner. For children with ASD, simultaneous demand for story construction and peer collaboration seems a complex endeavor due to their pragmatic difficulties. While the proposed technological interface may serve almost "on its own" to facilitate social interaction and play skills (27), results on story evaluation suggest that some steps should be taken to improve the quality of stories. These may include careful design of story backgrounds, more structured story prompts, and planned scaffolding protocols, where the technological interface could function as a facilitator within a thorough speech oriented program.

In summary, the findings of this study show the potential of the StoryTable to enhance authentic and creative storytelling among peers who share similar difficulties, as are children with ASD. More work is needed to corroborate these preliminary findings, investigating larger samples as well as other populations such as typically developing children and children with other developmental deficits. This will allow for a more comprehensive and reliable evaluation of the potential of technology to enhance communication and narrative abilities.

References

[1] Bruner JS. Actual minds, possible worlds. Cambridge, Ma: Harvard Univ. Press, 1986.

[2] Reilly J, Losh M, Bellugi U, Wulfeck B. "Frog, where are you?" narratives in children with specific language impairment, early focal brain injury, and Williams syndrome. Brain Lang. 2004;88(2):229-47.

[3] Ninio A, Snow CE. Pragmatic development: Essays in developmental science. Boulder, CO: Westview Press, 1996.

[4] Nelson K. Narrative, time and the emergence of the encultured self. Culture Psychol. 2000;6(2):183.

[5] Berman RA, Slobin DI. Relating events in narrative. A crosslinguistic developmental study. Hillsdale, NJ: Lawrence Erlbaum, 1994.

[6] Peterson C, McCabe A. Developmental psycholinguistics. Three ways of looking at a child's narrative. New York: Plenum, 1983.

[7] Loveland KA, McEvoy R, Tunali B, Kelley M. Narrative story telling in autism and down's syndrome. Br. J. Dev. Psychol. 1990;8:9-23.

[8] Capps L, Losh M, Thurber C. "The frog ate the bug and made his mouth sad": Narrative competence in children with autism. J. Abnorm. Child Psych. 2000;28(2):193-204.

[9] Tager-Flusberg H, Sullivan K. Attributing mental states to story characters: A comparison of narratives produced by autistic and mentally retarded individuals. Appl. Psycholinguist 1995;16(3): 241-56.

[10] Losh M, Capps L. Narrative ability in high-functioning children with autism or asperger's syndrome. J. Autism Dev. Disord. 2003;33(3): 239-51.

[11] Baron-Cohen S, Leslie AM, Frith U. Mechanical, behavioural and intentional understanding of picture stories in autistic children. Br. J. Dev. Psychol. 1986;4(1):113-25.

[12] Tager-Flusberg H. Autistic children's talk about psychological states: Deficits in the early acquisition of a theory of mind. Child Dev. 1992;63(1):161-72.

[13] Diehl JJ, Bennetto L, Young EC. Story recall and narrative coherence of high-functioning children with autism spectrum disorders. J. Abnorm. Child Psych. 2006;34(1):83-98.

[14] Bosseler A, Massaro DW. Development and evaluation of a computer-animated tutor for vocabulary and language learning in children with autism. J. Autism Dev. Disord. 2003;33(6):653-72.

[15] Heimann M, Nelson KE, Tjus T, Gillberg C. Increasing reading and communication skills in children with autism through an interactive multimedia computer program. J. Autism Dev. Disord. 1995;25(5): 459-80.

[16] Cassell J. Towards a model of technology and literacy development: Story listening systems. Appl Dev Psych 2004;25:75-105.

[17] Cassell J, Ryokai K. Making space for voice: Technologies to support children's fantasy and storytelling. Pers. Ubiquit. Comput. 2001;5(3): 169-90.

[18] Dautenhahn K, Werry I. Towards interactive robots in autism therapy: Background, motivation and challenges. Pragmatics Cogn 2004;12(1):1-35.

[19] Davis M, Dautenhahn K, Nehaniv CL, Powell SD. Towards an interactive system eliciting narrative comprehension in children with autism: A longitudinal study. In Clarkson J, Langdon P, Robinson P. Designing accessible technology. London: Springer, 2006:101-14.

[20] Hetzroni OE, Tannous J. Effects of a computer-based intervention program on the communicative functions of children with autism. J. Autism Dev. Disord. 2004;34(2):95-113.

[21] Pontecorvo C, Zucchermaglio C. A passage to literacy: learning in a social context. In Goodman Y. How children construct literacy. New York: Int. Reading Assoc., 1990:55-78.

[22] Hayes DS, Casey DM. Dyadic versus individual storytelling by preschool children. J Genet Psychol 2002;163(4):445-58.

[23] Schopler E, Reichler R, Renner B. The Childhood Autism Rating Scale (CARS). Los Angeles: Western Psychological Services, 1988.

[24] Lord C, Rutter M, LeCouteur, A. Autism diagnostic interview-revised: a revised version of a diagnostic interview for caregivers of individuals with possible pervasive developmental disorders. J. Autism Dev. Disord. 1994;19:185-212.

[25] Dietz P, Leigh D. DiamondTouch: A multi-user touch technology. Proceedings of the 14th Annual ACM Symposium on User Interface Software and Technology (UIST) 2001:219-26.
[26] Zancanaro M, Pianesi F, Stock O, Venuti P, et al. Children in the museum: an environment for collaborative storytelling. In: Stock O, Zancanaro M. PEACH: intelligent interfaces for museum visits, Cognitive Technologies Series. Berlin: Springer, 2007:165-84.
[27] Gal E, Bauminger N, Goren-Bar D, Pianesi F, et al. Enhancing social communication of children with high functioning autism through a co-located interface. Artif. Intell. Soc. 2009;24:75-84.
[28] Trabasso T, Secco T, van den Broek P. Causal cohesion and story coherence. In Mandl H, Stein NL, Trabasso T. Learning and comprehension of text. Hillsdale, NJ: Lawrence Erlbaum, 1984:83-111.
[29] Halliday MAK, Hasan R. Cohesion in spoken and written English. London: Longman, 1976.
[30] Peterson C, McCabe A. Linking children's connective use and narrative macrostructure. In McCabe A, Peterson C. Developing narrative structure. Hillsdale, NJ: Lawrence Erlbaum, 1991:29-55.
[31] Chang C. The development of autonomy in preschool mandarin Chinese-speaking children's play narratives. Narrat. Inq. 1998;8(1):77–111.
[32] Fivush R, Hazzard A, McDermott Sales J, Sarfati D, Brown T. Creating coherence out of chaos? children's narratives of emotionally positive and negative events. Appl. Cogn. Psychol. 2003;17(1):1-19.
[33] Hudson JA, Shapiro LR. From knowing to telling: The development of children's scripts, stories, and personal narratives. In McCabe A, Peterson C. Developing narrative structure. Hillsdale: Lawrence Erlbaum, 1991:89-136.
[34] Baker-Sennett J, Matusov E, Rogoff B. Sociocultural processes of creative planning in children's playcrafting. In Light P, Butterworth G. Context and cognition: Ways of learning and knowing. Hillsdale, NJ: Lawrence Erlbaum, 1992:93-114.
[35] Sawyer RK. Improvisation and narrative. Narrat Inq 2002;12(2):319-49.
[36] Liles BZ. Narrative ability in normal and language disordered children. J. Speech Hear Res. 1985;28:123-33.
[37] Liles BZ. Episode organization and cohesive conjunctives in narratives of children with and without language disorders. J. Speech Hear Res. 1987;30:185-96.
[38] Tager-Flusberg H. «Once upon a ribbit»: Stories narrated by autistic children. Br. J. Dev. Psychol. 1995;13:45-59.
[39] Wolf D, Hicks D. The voice within the narrative: The development of intertextuality in young children stories. Discourse Process 1989;12:329-51.

In: Understanding Autism Spectrum Disorder
Editors: Ditza A Zachor and Joav Merrick
ISBN: 978-1-62081-353-9

Chapter 10

Diagnostic outcomes in school age siblings of children with autism

***Ifat Gamliel Seidman*[1], *Nurit Yirmiya**[*1], *Raaya Alon*[1], *Noa Ben Yitzhak*[1], *Catherine Lord*[2] and *Marian Sigman*[3]**
[1]Department of Psychology and School of Education, Hebrew University of Jerusalem, Mount Scopus, Jerusalem, Israel
[2]University of Michigan Autism and Communication Disorders Center (UMACC), Ann Arbor, Michigan, US
[3]Departments of Psychiatry and Psychology, University of California Los Angeles, Los Angeles, CA, US

Abstract

Cumulative evidence for several personality traits reflecting a milder form of autistic characteristics among first-degree relatives of probands with autism has led to the concept of the broad autism phenotype (BAP). The present chapter aims to describe diagnostic outcomes of 34 school-age siblings of probands with autism (SIBS-A), aged 9 to 12 years, compared to 42 matched siblings of children with typical development (SIBS-TD). The diagnostic outcomes were derived from the Baby Siblings Research Consortium categorizations using the Autism Diagnostic Observation Schedule (ADOS), the Social Communication Questionnaire (SCQ), and standardized cognitive and language measures. Results indicated that about 38% of the SIBS-A group (n = 13) were identified with BAP-related difficulties (i.e., a SIBS-A-BAP subgroup), significantly surpassing the 7% of siblings identified with BAP-related difficulties in the SIBS-TD group. Interestingly, verbal IQ scores were significantly higher for the subgroup of SIBS-A-BAP compared to SIBS-A and SIBS-TD who were identified with typical development (SIBS-A-TD and SIBS-TD-TD, respectively). The current chapter presents developmental trajectories of these 13 SIBS-A-BAP as previously assessed longitudinally from ages 4 months to 7 years. Results support previous observation of an increase in

* Correspondence: Professor Nurit Yirmiya, PhD, Department of Psychology and School of Education, Hebrew University of Jerusalem, Mount Scopus, 91905 Jerusalem, Israel. E-mail: NYirmiya@gmail.com; NuritYirmiya@huji.ac.il

BAP-related difficulties in siblings after the preschool years. Results are discussed in relation to the developmental trajectories of the BAP in siblings of children with autism.

Introduction

Autism, a neurodevelopmental disorder characterized by impairments in social interaction, communication (verbal and nonverbal), and behavior (repetitive and stereotyped behaviors), has long been known to have a strong genetic involvement. Evidence from twin studies shows a much higher concordance rate for the disorder in monozygotic than in dizygotic twins. For example, Bailey et al (1) found no dizygotic pairs in their sample who were concordant for autism, in contrast to 60% of their monozygotic pairs. This finding indicates an heritability estimate of more than 90% (2). In family studies that measured prevalence of autism spectrum disorders (ASD) in siblings of autistic probands, about 5% of these siblings were diagnosed with ASD. This rate is much higher than the current 0.6% population base rate of autism (3). Despite this convincing evidence from twin and family studies, major autism susceptibility loci have not been detected to date. One current proposal is that many cases of autism represent a complex genetic disorder that involves several different genes, with each gene likely contributing differentially to particular components of the autistic spectrum (2)

The existence of a genetic component is reinforced by accumulating evidence among relatives of autistic probands for a number of subtle personality, social, and language features that reflect a milder form of autism core characteristics. This more subtle form of ASD characteristics is referred to as the "broad autism phenotype" (BAP). The BAP was described by Bolton et al in 1994 (4) as a dysfunction in one or more of the three dysfunction domains of autism. Yet with time, specific elements other than those belonging to the triad of autism deficits were proposed as additional components of the BAP. The study of BAP characteristics is also the study of autism endophenotypes, which are variables that correlate with a given disease, are usually sub-clinical, involve fewer genes than those involved in the disease syndrome itself, and could assist in the identification of genes conferring vulnerability to the disorder. To meet the criteria for an endophenotype, a marker must be present in affected individuals, has to be heritable and co-segregate with the illness, should be state-independent (i.e., manifests in an individual whether or not the illness is active), and must be found among unaffected relatives of patients at a higher rate than in the general population (5,6).

One approach to investigating the BAP in siblings of children with autism (SIBS-A) is through interviews or questionnaires completed by an informant (usually a parent or teacher) regarding the unaffected sibling. These instruments include a pool of items measuring BAP-related traits, mainly pertaining to the triad of autism deficits. Using this approach with the Family History Interview has identified deficits in social or communication functioning in as many as 7% to 20% of SIBS-A (depending on the strictness of the definition used) (4,7). Virkud et al (8) employed the Social Responsiveness Scale (9), which focuses primarily on reciprocal social interaction and communication but includes some items inquiring about restricted and stereotypic behaviors or interests as well. This scale revealed elevated scores for SIBS-A in comparison to siblings of probands with psychopathology unrelated to autism. Additional recent instruments of this kind include the Broader Phenotype Autism Symptom

Scale (BPASS; 10) and the Broad Autism Phenotype Questionnaire (BAPQ) (11), but these scales have thus far been used only for investigating BAP in parents, not in siblings.

Several specific candidate traits for the BAP have been investigated in siblings: executive functions like cognitive flexibility, planning, inhibition, set-shifting, generativity, and working memory (6,12,13); externalizing and internalizing behavior problems (14,15); learning disabilities (16); theory of mind (17); general cognitive abilities (13,16,18,19), and a range of lingual aspects (16,18,20-23).

In the current study, we examined BAP-related difficulties using the Autism Diagnostic Observation Schedule (ADOS; 24), in SIBS-A aged 9-12 years. The ADOS is a well-known diagnostic system for ASD. It provides several activities and tasks to enable evaluation of social, communicative, and behavioral functioning. Examining siblings at school age is important because it allows observation of features that characterize SIBS-A at a relatively late stage in the course of development, features that perhaps cannot be observed in earlier ages. To the best of our knowledge, the ADOS has not yet been administered to SIBS-A of this age group with the purpose of identifying the BAP. In addition to using the ADOS, which refers to the triad of autism deficits, we also assessed linguistic and cognitive abilities hypothesized as BAP-related.

Research on cognitive abilities in SIBS-A has yielded inconsistent outcomes. Some studies comparing cognitive ability indices of SIBS-A with siblings of children with typical development (SIBS-TD) or with siblings of children with other developmental disorders reported higher rates of cognitive delays (16) or lower performance on IQ tests (19) for the SIBS-A, whereas others reported no such differences (13,18).

Studies of language abilities in SIBS-A also had inconsistent findings. Some researchers found that SIBS-A performed lower on such tests (16) and demonstrated higher rates of language difficulties compared to a comparison group (20). Other research using language indices showed no significant performance differences between SIBS-A and a comparison group or the test norms (18, 23) or even better performance by the SIBS-A (22).

Variability in findings regarding cognitive and linguistic abilities of SIBS-A may be partially due to age variability between and within samples of different studies. As linguistic and cognitive abilities are developmental in nature, age is a critical methodological issue. The current follow-up research is part of a longitudinal study following a sample of SIBS-A and SIBS-TD from infancy to childhood. So far, these children were seen at the ages of 4, 14, 24, 36, 54 months, 7 years, and now at 9-12 years. The relative homogeneity of ages in our sample, as well as the use of a comparison group that was well-matched at the beginning of the study, have so far enabled us to observe subtle differences between the two groups.

In the first five time points, we examined aspects of linguistic and cognitive delays, defined as scores of at least two SDs below average on the cognitive and/or language measures. During their first 24 months of life, 12 out of the 39 SIBS-A in our sample were identified as having language and/or cognitive delays (including 1 child later diagnosed with autism). This rate of delays was significantly higher than in the SIBS-TD group, where only 2 out of the 39 children manifested such delays. These data indicate that most SIBS-A developed well in terms of cognition and language through toddlerhood. Moreover, most of the differences that were observed up to age 36 months disappeared at 54 months, with the exception of continued lower expressive language scores in SIBS-A compared to SIBS-TD (25). At 7 years, in addition to examining linguistic and cognitive delays by means of standardized measures (this time defining a delay as scores at least 1.5 SD below average), we also collected a parental report regarding school-related difficulties (an adaptation of the Family History Interview). Results showed that 15 out of 37 SIBS-A at age 7 revealed BAP-related difficulties according to cognitive and language measures and/or parental reports, comprising significantly more than the 6 out of 37 SIBS-TD who manifested such difficulties (26).

The current study aims to further describe the developmental trajectories of this sample of SIBS-A and SIBS-TD, now aged 9-12 years. This time, in addition to the administration of language and intelligence tests, we also administered the ADOS and used an adaptation of the Baby Siblings Research Consortium (BSRC) to classify diagnostic outcomes based on studies of SIBS-A (27).

The Consortium classification of the BAP is determined by the child's performance on the ADOS assessment. After classifying each sibling as fitting or not fitting BAP criteria, we examined the cognitive and language aspects hypothesized as BAP-related by comparing the three groups' performance on standardized indices (SIBS-A with BAP, SIBS-A without BAP, SIBS-TD). We hypothesized that more SIBS-A would be diagnosed with the BAP compared to the SIBS-TD. Given past findings of significant as well as nonsignificant differences among SIBS-A and SIBS-TD in language and cognition, we did not state specific hypotheses for possible differences in these areas among SIBS-A with BAP, SIBS-A without BAP, and SIBS-TD.

Our study

The SIBS-A group comprises 34 children (11 girls/23 boys) having an older sibling with autism. The participants took part in our longitudinal study on the development of siblings of children with autism and were previously seen at the ages of 4, 14, 24, 36, and 54 months, and at 7 years. At the current assessment, the age of the SIBS-A ranged from 8 years/11 months to 12 years/1 month (M = 10 years/1 month; SD = 9.21 months).

The older siblings, the probands with autism (8 girls/¬25 boys - two of the siblings had the same proband), had a previous diagnosis of autism made by independent clinicians before our study. However, for the purpose of the present study, diagnosis of autism was confirmed by two independent clinicians, blind to all other study procedures, using the Autism Diagnostic Observation Schedule-Generic (ADOS-G) (28) and/or the Autism Diagnostic Interview-Revised (ADI-R) (29). Some of the probands were recruited before the availability of the ADOS-G in Israel and therefore were administered only the ADI-R. Parents were interviewed using the ADI-R and the Vineland Adaptive Behavior Scale-Interview Edition (VABS) (30) regarding the proband with autism.

The probands' IQ was measured with a standard IQ test appropriate to age and/or developmental ability, i.e., Bayley Scales of Infant Development-2nd edition (31); Kaufman Assessment Battery for Children (32), or Wechsler Intelligence Scale for Children-3rd edition (33). Based on these tests, 8 of the 33 probands were classified as high functioning (IQ and/or daily living skills score > 70), whereas the remaining 25 probands were classified as low functioning (IQ and daily living skills score < 70).

Inclusion criteria for families in this group were: (a) intact families who had a child with autism and a younger sibling; (b) normal pregnancy with the participating sibling as reported by the parents, with no peri-, pre-, or post-natal difficulties as well as normal gestational age (>36 weeks); and (c) no medical conditions associated with autism such as Fragile X or tuberous sclerosis in the proband. The families were recruited through treatment centers, special schools, the Israeli national organization for children with autism, and families of children with autism.

The SIBS-TD group and matching procedure. The comparison group comprised 42 siblings (21 girls/21 boys) of typically developing children. The ages of SIBS-TD ranged from 9 years/1 month to 12 years/1 month (M = 9 years/9 months; SD = 9.45 months), with no significant difference emerging in age between the two groups ($t(1, 74) = 1.67$, $p = .10$, $d = .39$). Families in this SIBS-TD group were recruited from maternity wards in Jerusalem. Inclusion criteria required that: (a) the families were intact at the time of the study's initiation; (b) the older child exhibited typical development with no history of any medical, learning, and/or emotional difficulties and had not received any specialized interventions such as occupational therapy, speech and language therapy, or psychotherapy based on parental report; and (c) the pregnancy with the participating sibling was normal as reported by the parents.

The two groups were matched at 4 months on a one-to one basis according to chronological age (CA), sex, birth order, number of children in the family, sex of the older proband, temperament profile (ICQ: Infant Characteristics Questionnaire) (34), and Bayley (31) mental and motor scores. SIBS-A who joined the study after the age of 4 months were matched to SIBS-TD according to the same variables, as best as possible. Parents' age, ethnicity, income, and education level did not significantly differ between the two groups at the age of 4 months. At each age, we reexamined these background variables and found no significant differences between the groups. Attrition rate was very low. Only three siblings from the SIBS-A group were not tested: One family relocated outside of Israel, one was unwilling to participate, and one could not be found.

Measures

Autism Diagnostic Observation Schedule (ADOS) (24). The ADOS, one of the gold-standard diagnostic systems for ASD, is a semi-structured, standardized observational assessment designed to assess behaviors related to autism or ASD, based on the DSM-IV (35) and the ICD-10 (36) criteria for ASD. It provides several opportunities for communication, social interaction, and play or imaginative use of materials, and includes social, communicative, and behavioral measures diagnostic of autism.

The ADOS consists of four modules designated for use according to chronological age, language, and cognitive abilities. In the current study of children aged 9-12 years, Module 4 was administered to all participants. To determine cutoff scores for "autism" and "ASD" classifications on the ADOS, an algorithm is calculated based on a subset of items. In the current study, we used the revised algorithm published by Gotham et al (37), which includes the Social Affect and the Restricted Repetitive Behaviors domains. Although revised algorithms were published only for Modules 1-3, we were able to use the algorithm published for Module 3 for children who received Module 4 because all of the Module 3 items overlapped were also in Module 4.

Because the study was carried out in participants' homes, it was impossible at times to conceal the group identity of the participant (e.g., the older sibling with autism was at home). Therefore, the ADOS administration was videotaped and coded later by 2 of 3 coders who were blind to group assignment. Inter-rater reliability was assessed for 59 administrations and yielded 91.47% agreement among the 3 coders. The Social Communication Questionnaire (SCQ) (38). The SCQ, which includes 40-items and is based on items from the ADI-R (29), was designed as a screening instrument for caregivers of children 4 years and older to evaluate autism spectrum symptoms. The SCQ has good discriminative validity with respect to the separation of ASD from non-ASD diagnoses at all IQ levels (39). In line with Corsello et al (40), we used a cutoff of 11 in addition to the ADOS. Wechsler Intelligence Scale for Children (WISC-III) (33). The WISC-III is a standardized test designed to assess intellectual abilities of children between the ages of 6-16 years. Subtest scores are combined to provide scaled scores for Verbal IQ (VIQ), Performance IQ (PIQ), and Full Scale IQ (FSIQ). Clinical Evaluation of Language Fundamentals – 3rd edition (CELF-III; (41). The CELF-III is a standardized test designed to assess a wide range of language abilities of individuals between the ages of 6 and 21 years. Its subtest scores are summed into two scales, receptive language ability and expressive language ability, and combined into a total language score. Demographic information. Background details including the number of children, family income, parents' employment status, and parents' education were collected.

Procedure

Families were contacted and invited to participate in the study. Each sibling was seen individually for three videotaped sessions. The WISC-III IQ test and the CELF-III language test were administered by the same experimenter during the first two sessions, each lasting about 120 minutes. In the third session, which lasted about 60 minutes, the ADOS was administered by a different experimenter. Each experimenter was blind to participants' performance on the other measures and the order of the WISC and CELF III sessions was randomly assigned for the two groups. Parents completed the SCQ and the demographic questionnaires. Evaluation procedures were compatible with children's attention span and activity level. Breaks were given as often as needed. Parents received a detailed report summarizing their child's performance upon completion.

Our findings

SIBS-A, aged 9 to 12 years, were classified into diagnostic outcome categories using an adaptation of the BSRC classifications from studies of SIBS-A (27).

These criteria, which are presented in table 1, include seven categories: Autism, ASD, General Developmental Delay (GDD), Language Delay (LD), BAP Difficulties, Typical Development (TD) and other.

Table 1. Siblings of children with autism (SIBS-A) and siblings of children with typical development (SIBS-TD): Outcome categories

Category	SIBS-A ($n = 34$)	SIBS-TD ($n = 42$)	Criteria
Autism	$n = 0$	$n = 0$	1. Above Autism cutoff on ADOS (Module 4); and 2. Above Autism cutoff on SCQ; and 3. Meets *DSM-IV* criteria for Autistic Disorder.
Autism Spectrum Disorders (ASD)	$n = 1$	$n = 0$	1. Above ASD cutoff on ADOS (Module 4); and 2. Above ASD cutoff on SCQ; and 3. Meets *DSM-IV* criteria for PDD-NOS; and 4. Does not meet criteria for Autism.
General Developmental Delay (GDD)	$n = 1$	$n = 0$	1. WISC Full IQ ≤ 78; and 2. At least one WISC performance subtest ≤ 5; and 3. CELF receptive or CELF expressive ≤ 78; and 4. Does not meet criteria for ASD or Autism.
Language Delay (LD)	$n = 0$	$n = 0$	1. CELF receptive or CELF expressive ≤ 70; or CELF receptive and CELF expressive ≤ 78; and 2. Does not meet criteria for GDD, ASD, or Autism.
BAP Difficulties	$n = 13$	$n = 3$	1. ADOS score (Module 4) ≥ 4; and 2. Does not meet criteria for LD, GDD, ASD, or Autism.
Typical Development (TD)	$n = 19$	$n = 38$	1. WISC Full IQ, and Verbal IQ, and Performance IQ, and CELF receptive, and CELF expressive > 70; and 2. No more than one score ≤ 78 on the WISC Full IQ, Verbal IQ, Performance IQ, CELF receptive, or CELF expressive; and 3. Does not meet criteria for BAP Difficulties, LD, GDD, ASD, or Autism.
Other	$n = 0$	$n = 1$	Does not meet criteria for any of the above classifications

The number of siblings assigned to each category is also presented in table 1. Among the SIBS-A group, 1 sibling was diagnosed with ASD (in line with his previous diagnosis of ASD from previous time points); 1 sibling was identified with GDD; 13 siblings were identified with BAP-related difficulties; and 19 siblings were identified with TD. Among the SIBS-TD group, none of the siblings was identified with Autism, ASD, GDD, or LD; 3 siblings were identified with BAP-related difficulties; 38 siblings were identified with TD; and 1 sibling was identified as Other. Thus, in the SIBS-A group, 13 out of 34 siblings (38.24%) were identified with BAP-related difficulties, in contrast to 3 out of 42 (7.14%) siblings in the SIBS-TD group. This difference was significant, $\chi^2_{(1/76)} = 10.93$, $p = .001$. Current diagnostic, cognition, and language data of siblings identified with BAP-related difficulties in both groups are presented in table 2. We also examined the developmental histories (at the previous time points of our longitudinal study) (25,26,42,43) of the subgroup of siblings who were currently identified with BAP-related difficulties. Interestingly, 9 of the 13 SIBS-A (69.23%) who were currently identified with BAP-related difficulties had also been previously identified with BAP-related difficulties (e.g., at age 14, 24, 36, or 54 months or 7 years), whereas only 1 of the 3 SIBS-TD who were currently identified with BAP-related difficulties had been previously identified. Specifically, within the SIBS-A group (see table 2), Sibling B was identified with language delay at age 14 months but not later; Sibling L was identified with cognitive and language delays at 24 and 36 months but not later; Sibling I was first identified with language delay at age 24 months and with later cognitive and/or language difficulties at age 7 years; and Siblings C, E, G, H, J, and M were first identified with cognitive and/or language difficulties at age 7 years. Within the SIBS-TD group (table 2), only Sibling N was previously identified with cognitive and/or language difficulties at age 7 years.

Intergroup analyses: Cognitive and language scores

Analyses of variance were employed to compare the cognitive and language abilities of the three groups: SIBS-A identified with BAP-related difficulties (i.e., SIBS-A-BAP, n = 13); SIBS-A identified with TD (SIBS-A-TD, n = 19); and SIBS-TD identified with TD (SIBS-TD-TD, n = 38). These data are presented in table 3. In addition to significant findings based on group comparisons, we also examined effect sizes, which are independent of sample size. Following Cohen (44), an effect size of d = .80 indicates a nonoverlap of almost 50% in the two distributions and is considered as large. Thus, we only interpreted effect sizes of .80 and above. Regarding cognition scores, analyses of variance revealed no significant overall group effect for the Verbal IQ and the Performance IQ among the three groups (F (4, 130) = 1.38, $p = .25$, $\eta_p^2 = .04$). However, a near-significant group effect was yielded for the Verbal IQ score ($F_{(2,\ 66)} = 2.64$, $p = .08$, $\eta_p^2 = .07$). As seen in table 3, Fisher's least significant difference (LSD) post-hoc tests revealed that as a group, SIBS-A-BAP tended to have a significantly higher Verbal IQ score (M = 115.46, SD = 15.13) than SIBS-TD-TD (M = 106.32, SD = 11; p = .03, d = .69). No other significant differences or large effect sizes were yielded for the LSD post-hoc comparisons, either between the SIBS-A-TD group and the SIBS-A-BAP group or between the SIBS-A-TD group and the SIBS-TD-TD group (table 3).

Table 2. Current data on sibling subgroup classified with broad autism phenotype (BAP)

ID	Sex	Diagnostic scores		Cognition (IQ) scores			Language (CELF) scores	
		ADOS	SCQ	Full	Verbal	Performance	Receptive	Expressive
SIBS-A ($n = 13$)								
A	F	7	0	109	119	98	131	128
B	M	7	1	101	113	87	114	112
C	M	7	0	120	118	117	120	114
D	F	4	5	115	118	110	131	128
E	M	4	7	123	117	127	143	110
F	F	6	1	115	122	106	128	114
G	M	17	3	85	91	81	90	94
H	M	6	5	111	118	102	108	104
I	M	5	3	121	129	107	116	108
J	M	6	2	134	148	113	114	102
K	M	4	-	109	117	99	-	-
L	M	10	-	104	92	106	102	90
M	M	10	4	90	99	82	116	98
SIBS-TD ($n = 3$)								
N	M	7	6	83	91	78	82	90
O	M	6	9	83	93	74	94	98
P	F	6	-	93	87	103	92	80

Table 3. Group comparisons between the three groups on cognition (IQ) and language (CELF)

		SIBS-A-BAP (n = 13)	SIBS-A-TD (n = 19)	SIBS-TD-TD (n = 38)	Post-hoc LSD	p	Effect size (d)
Verbal IQ	*M*	115.46	109.95	106.32	SIBS-A-BAP = SIBS-A-TD	.23	.39
	(*SD*)	(15.13)	(13.38)	(11.00)	SIBS-A-BAP > SIBS-TD-TD	.03*	.69
					SIBS-A-TD = SIBS-TD-TD	.31	.30
Performance IQ	*M*	102.69	101.42	101.41	SIBS-A-BAP = SIBS-A-TD	.75	.11
	(*SD*)	(13.47)	(9.33)	(10.47)	SIBS-A-BAP = SIBS-TD-TD	.71	.11
					SIBS-A-TD = SIBS-TD-TD	.99	.00
CELF Receptive	*M*	117.75	115.37	112.29	SIBS-A-BAP = SIBS-A-TD	.65	.16
	(*SD*)	(14.29)	(14.91)	(13.45)	SIBS-A-BAP = SIBS-TD-TD	.24	.39
					SIBS-A-TD = SIBS-TD-TD	.44	.22
CELF Expressive	*M*	108.5	106.32	103.53	SIBS-A-BAP = SIBS-A-TD	.59	.19
	(*SD*)	(11.91)	(11.28)	(10.53)	SIBS-A-BAP = SIBS-TD-TD	.18	.44
					SIBS-A-TD = SIBS-TD-TD	.37	.26

* $p < .05$.

Regarding language scores (CELF Receptive and Expressive scores), analyses of variance revealed no significant overall group effect for the two language scores ($F_{(4, 130)}$ = .62, p = .65, η_p^2 = .02), as well as no significant group differences or large effect sizes for the LSD post-hoc tests (table 3).

Discussion

The BAP-related difficulties of school-age SIBS-A were compared to those of SIBS-TD based on an adaptation of the BSRC classifications (27). Using the ADOS, the SCQ, and cognitive and language tests, a subgroup of 13 children from the SIBS-A group (SIBS-A-BAP) was identified, compared to only three children identified from the SIBS-TD group. Thus, compared to SIBS-TD, significantly more SIBS-A were identified with BAP-related difficulties, i.e., elevated ADOS scores as well as IQ and language scores within the normative range, according to the BSRC criteria. These findings regarding the BAP rate (38%) were similar to our previous findings at age 7 years (about 40%; see 26), thus supporting the observation of an increase in BAP-related difficulties in siblings after the preschool years, when the BAP rate was about 28% (25,42,43).

Several explanations may be suggested. First, it is possible that BAP-related difficulties are more subtle and not yet noticeable during the first years of life, thus suggesting a "sleeper effect" kind of trajectory, or different underlying mechanisms in toddlerhood compared to later childhood development, as recently suggested by Rogers (45) to explain the lack of overt behavioral identifiers or early markers of ASD before age 12 months. Another possible explanation may be that screeners and diagnostic measures in the preschool years are not sensitive enough to detect BAP-related difficulties or ASD symptoms in less impaired toddlers, who may not show marked deficits in the development of communication and social behaviors (45). Furthermore, in our prospective study differences in BAP rates may be attributed to the additional measures used for detecting BAP difficulties at school age (e.g., ADOS, parent reports), beyond the cognitive and language tests used both in the preschool and the school years. Thus, our longitudinal cohort's increase in the rate of BAP difficulties during the school years may reflect either a discontinuity in developmental trajectories of BAP or better sensitivity of measures after the preschool years or both.

The findings regarding school age BAP difficulties in social, communicative, and behavioral adjustment that emerged in this study using the ADOS, a well-known diagnostic measure for ASD, coincide with other studies that yielded difficulties in the triad of autism (1,4,7). For example, researchers addressing social and emotional adjustment of SIBS-A, as part of the BAP, reported increased rates of behavior and adjustment problems including impaired social play and conversation, aggressive behavior, limited relationships, and social inappropriateness among SIBS-A compared to SIBS-TD and siblings of children with mental retardation (8,14,15,46,47). However, other researchers found that SIBS-A were well adjusted compared to siblings of children with other disabilities or compared to SIBS-TD (48,49,50). As previously suggested, some of the contradictions in the literature may be attributed to methodological issues such as using different assessment methods, comparison groups, and participant ages. Our findings support evidence for BAP difficulties among a subgroup of

SIBS-A, whereas the rest of the SIBS-A manifested typical and adjusted social development in school age as measured using the ADOS.

The developmental histories of the 13 SIBS-A-BAP yielded interesting findings. Almost 70% of the children in the SIBS-A-BAP subgroup were previously identified at 14, 24, 36, or 54 months or at 7 years (25,26,42,43). These findings suggest several different trajectories for the development of BAP among siblings. Some of the difficulties are continuous, some are transient, and others appear for the first time during the school years. It seems that the different trajectories may be associated both with individual differences as well as with developmental milestones characteristic to each period and also with significant plasticity in their course of development. Thus, the following questions may arise: Are some of the BAP-related difficulties genuinely resolved during development? If so, should intervention be recommended anyway for those BAP siblings?

Another interesting finding in this study is that as a group the SIBS-A-BAP had higher Verbal IQ scores than the other two groups of SIBS-A-TD and SIBS-TD-TD. Similarly, Fombonne (19) and Pilowsky (22) found that SIBS-A performed better on tests of verbal ability than did siblings of children with developmental language delays and siblings of children with Down syndrome. This result may reflect that this subgroup of SIBS-A children identified with BAP difficulties on the ADOS are compensating for their social, communication, and behavioral difficulties with better language abilities. An alternative explanation may be that their higher verbal abilities could be associated with difficulties in pragmatic language (i.e., inappropriate formal language or prolonged conversations), which are measured in the ADOS and considered part of the BAP (18).

Study limitations include the relatively small sample size and the resulting small subgroups, as well as the lack of other comparison groups (i.e., siblings of children with other disabilities such as mental retardation or language delays). However, using a comparison group of SIBS-TD provided normative data as a basis of comparison for the development of SIBS-A. This comparison thus enabled the exploration of whether SIBS-A as a group demonstrated subtle impairments compared to the SIBS-TD, or whether some SIBS-A appeared to develop typically while others seemed significantly affected (i.e., SIBS-A-BAP).

Finally, the investigation of BAP in siblings of probands with ASD is one of enormous importance to enhance parents', caregivers', and professionals' awareness about these siblings' risk for developing deficits in various domains of function, which can lead to earlier and more effective interventions. Our data suggests that siblings may need regular assessments and observations even into the school years and not only during infancy. At the same time, as demonstrated in our longitudinal study, some of the siblings are developing well and some of their difficulties were transient; therefore, the current study also underscores the importance of educating parents and professionals regarding these possibilities as well.

Acknowledgments

This study was supported by the United States-Israel Binational Science Foundation (BSF), Grant # 2007209, awarded to NY, MS, and CL. We are grateful to the families who took part for their cooperation and to Dee B. Ankonina for her editorial assistance.

References

[1] Bailey A, Le Couteur A, Gottesman I, Bolton P, Simonoff E, Yuzda E, et al. Autism as a strongly genetic disorder: evidence from a British twin study. Psychol. Med. 1995;25:63-77.

[2] Folstein S, Rosen-Sheidley B. Genetics of austim: complex aetiology for a heterogeneous disorder. Nat. Rev. Genet. 2001;2:943-55.

[3] Szatmari P, Jones M, Zwaigenbaum L, MacLean J. Genetics of autism: overview and new directions. J. Autism Dev. Disord. 1998;28:351-68.

[4] Bolton P, Macdonald H, Pickles A, Rios P, Goode S, Crowson M, et al. A case-control family history study of autism. J. Child Psychol. Psychiatry 1994;35:877-900.

[5] Gottesman I, Gould T. The endophenotype concept in psychiatry: etymology and strategic intentions. Am. Psychiatric Assoc. 2003;160:636-45.

[6] Delorme R, Gouss V, Roy I, Trandafir A, Mathieu F, Mouren-Simoni M, et al. Shared executive dysfunctions in unaffected relatives of patients with autism and obsessive-compulsive disorder. Eur. Psychiatry 2007;22:32-8.

[7] Pickles A, Starr E, Kazak S, Bolton P, Papanikolaou K, Bailey A, et al. Variable expression of the autism broader phenotype: findings from extended pedigrees. J. Child Psychol. Psychiatry 2000;41:491-502.

[8] Virkud Y, Todd R, Abbacchi, A, Zhang Y, Constantino J. Familial aggregation of quantitative autistic traits in multiplex versus simplex autism. Am. J. Med. Genet. Part B 2008;150B:328-34.

[9] Constantino J, Przybeck T, Friesen D, Todd R. Reciprocal social behavior in children with and without pervasive developmental disorders. J. Dev. Behav. Pediatr. 2000;21:2-11.

[10] Dawson G, Estes A, Munson J, Schellenberg G, Bernier R, Abbott R. Quantitative assessment of autism symptom-related traits in probands and parents: broader phenotype autism symptom scale. J. Autism Dev. Disord 2007;37:523-36.

[11] Hurley R, Losh M, Parlier M, Reznick J, Piven J. The broad autism phenotype questionnaire. J. Autism Dev. Disord. 2007;37:1679-90.

[12] Wong D, Maybery M, Bishop D, Maley A, Hallmayer J. Profiles of executive function in parents and siblings of individuals with autism spectrum disorders. Genes. Brain Behav. 2006;5:561-76.

[13] Pilowsky T, Yirmiya, N, Shalev, R, and Gross-Tzur, V. Neuropsychological functioning of siblings of children with autism, siblings of children with developmental language delay, and siblings of children with mental retardation of unknown genetic etiology. J. Autism Dev. Disord. 2007;37:537-52.

[14] Fisman S, Wolf L, Ellison D, Gillis B, Freeman T, Szatmari P. Risk and protective factors affecting the adjustment of siblings of children with chronic disabilities. J Am Acad Child Adol Psychiatry 1996;35:1532-41.

[15] Gold N. Depression and social adjustment in siblings of boys with autism. J. Autism Dev. Disord. 1993;23:147-63.

[16] August G, Stewart M, Tsai L. The incidence of cognitive disabilities in the siblings of autistic children. Brit. J. Psychiatry 1981;138:416-22.

[17] Shaked M, Gamliel I, Yirmiya N. Theory of mind abilities in young siblings of children with autism. Autism 2006;10:173-87.

[18] Folstein S, Santangelo S, Gilman S, Piven J, Landa R, Lainhart J, et al. Predictors of cognitive test patterns in autism families. J. Child Psychol. Psychiatry 1999;40:1117-28.

[19] Fombonne E, Bolton P, Prior J, Jordan H, Rutter M. A family study of autism: cognitive patterns and levels in parents and siblings. J. Child Psychol. Psychiatry 1997;38:667-83.

[20] Chuthapisith J, Ruangdaraganon N, Sombuntham T, Roongpraiwan R. Language development among the siblings of children with autistic spectrum disorder. Autism 2007;11:149-160.

[21] Le Couteur A, Bailey A, Goode S, Pickles A, Robertson S, Gottesman I, et al. A broader phenotype of autism: the clinical spectrum in twins. J. Child. Psychol. Psychiatry 1996;37:785-802.

[22] Pilowsky T, Yirmiya N, Shalev R, Gross-Tsur V. Language abilities of siblings of children with autism. J. Child Psychol. Psychiatry 2003;44:914-25.

[23] Smalley S, Asarnow R. Brief report: Cognitive subclinical markers in autism. J. Autism Dev. Disord. 1990;20:271-8.

[24] Lord C, Rutter M, DiLavore P, Risi S. Autism diagnostic observation schedule. Los Angeles, CA: Western Psychol. Serv, 2002.
[25] Gamliel I, Yirmiya N, Sigman M. The development of young siblings of children with autism from 4 to 54 months. J. Autism Dev. Disord. 2007;37:171-83.
[26] Gamliel I, Yirmiya N, Jaffe D, Manor O, Sigman M. Developmental trajectories in siblings of children with autism: cognition and language from 4 months to 7 years. J. Autism Dev. Disord. 2009;39:1131-44.
[27] Ozonoff S, Macari S, Young G, Goldring S, Thompson M, Rogers S. Atypical object exploration at 12 months of age is associated with autism in a prospective sample. Autism 2008;12:457-72.
[28] Lord C, Risi S, Lambrecht L, Cook E, Leventhal B, DiLavore P, et al. The autism diagnostic observation schedule-generic: A standard measure of social and communication deficits associated with the spectrum of autism. J. Autism Dev. Disord. 2000;30:205-23.
[29] Lord C, Rutter M, Couteur A. Autism diagnostic interview-revised: a revised version of a diagnostic interview for caregivers of individuals with possible pervasive developmental disorders. J. Autism Dev. Disord. 1994;24:659-85.
[30] Sparrow SS, Balla, DA, Cicchetti, DV. Vineland adaptive behavior scales. Circle Pines, MN: Am. Guidance Serv., 1985.
[31] Bayley N. Bayley scales of infant development. New York: Psychol. Corp, 1993.
[32] Kaufman AS, Kaufman, NL. Kaufman assessment battery for children (K-ABC). Circle Pines, MN: Am. Guidance Serv., 1983.
[33] Wechsler D. Wechsler intelligence scale for children. San Antonio, TX: Psychol. Corp., 1991.
[34] Bates J, Freeland C, Lounsbury M. Measurement of infant difficultness. Child Dev. 1979;50:794-803.
[35] American Psychiatric Association. Diagnostic and statistical manual of mental disorders (4th ed.). Washington, DC: Author, 1994.
[36] World Health Organization. The ICD-10 classification of mental and behavioural disorders: clinical descriptions and diagnostic guidelines. Geneva: Author, 1992.
[37] Gotham K, Risi S, Pickles A, Lord C. The autism diagnostic observation schedule: revised algorithms for improved diagnostic validity. J. Autism Dev. Disord. 2007;37:613-27.
[38] Rutter M, Bailey A, Lord C, Berument S. Social communication questionnaire. Los Angeles: Western Psychol. Serv., 2003.
[39] Berument S, Rutter M, Lord C, Pickles A, Bailey A. Autism screening questionnaire: diagnostic validity. Br. J. Psychiatry 1999;175:444-51.
[40] Corsello C, Hus V, Pickles A, Risi S, Cook E, Leventhal B, et al. Between a ROC and a hard place: decision making and making decisions about using the SCQ. J. Child Psychol. Psychiatry 2007;48:932-40.
[41] Semel E, Wiig, EH, Secord, WA. Clinical evaluation and language fundamentals (CELF) (3rd ed.). San Antonio: Psychol. Corp./Harcourt Brace, 1995.
[42] Yirmiya N, Gamliel I, Pilowsky T, Feldman R, Baron-Cohen S, Sigman M. The development of siblings of children with autism at 4 and 14 months: social engagement, communication, and cognition. J. Child Psychol. Psychiatry 2006;47:511-23.
[43] Yirmiya N, Gamliel I, Shaked M, Sigman M. Cognitive and verbal abilities of 24-to 36-month-old siblings of children with autism. J. Autism Dev. Disord. 2007;37:218-29.
[44] Cohen J. Statistical power analysis for the behavioral sciences. Hillsdale, NJ: Lawrence Erlbaum, 1988.
[45] Rogers S. What are infant siblings teaching us about autism in infancy? Autism Res. 2009;2:125-37.
[46] Macks R, Reeve R. The adjustment of non-disabled siblings of children with autism. J. Autism Dev. Disord. 2007;37:1060-7.
[47] Piven J, Palmer P, Jacobi D, Childress D, Arndt S. Broader autism phenotype: evidence from a family history study of multiple-incidence autism families. Am. Psychiatric Assoc. 1997;154:185-90.
[48] Happe F, Frith U, Briskman J. Exploring the cognitive phenotype of autism: weak "central coherence" in parents and siblings of children with autism: I. Experimental tests. J. Child Psychol. Psychiatry 2001;42:299-307.

[49] Pilowsky T, Yirmiya N, Doppelt O, Gross-Tsur V, Shalev R. Social and emotional adjustment of siblings of children with autism. J. Child Psychol. Psychiatry 2004;45:855-65.

[50] Verte S, Roeyers H, Buysse A. Behavioural problems, social competence and self-concept in siblings of children with autism. Child Care Health Dev. 2003;29:193-205.

In: Understanding Autism Spectrum Disorder
Editors: Ditza A Zachor and Joav Merrick
ISBN: 978-1-62081-353-9

Chapter 11

Safety and efficacy of donepezil in children and adolescents with autism: Behavioral measures

Benjamin L Handen*, Cynthia R Johnson, Sarah McAuliffe-Bellin and Antonio Hardan
Western Psychiatric Institute and Clinic and Children's Hospital of Pittsburgh, University of Pittsburgh School of Medicine, Pittsburgh, Pennsylvania and Department of Psychiatry and Behavioral Sciences, Stanford University, Stanford, California, US

Abstract

The desire to ameliorate behavioral, social and communication deficits in Autism Spectrum Disorder (ASD) has led to increased interest in the use of cognitive enhancing drugs, such as cholinesterase inhibitors, as a possible treatment for ASD.

Objective: The objective of the current study was to assess the tolerability, safety and efficacy of donepezil on behavioral functioning in a group of children and adolescents with ASD. Study Group: A group of 34 children and adolescents (ages 8-17 years; IQ>75) with ASD were enrolled in the study.

Methods: The study involved a 10-week, double-blind, placebo-controlled trial of donepezil (doses of 5 mg and 10 mg), followed by a 10-week open label trial for placebo non-responders.

Results and Conclusions: The current chapter summarizes the results of a set of behavioral outcome measures. While gains were noted across a number of dependent measures of behavior and core features of autism, improvement was noted for both the placebo and active medication groups. No statistically significant between groups differences were found. The results reinforce the need to conduct well-controlled treatment outcome trials in ASD.

---

* Correspondence: Benjamin L Handen, PhD, Western Psychiatric Institute and Clinic, 1011 Bingham St, Pittsburgh, PA 15203 United States. E-mail: handenbl@upmc.edu

Introduction

Autism spectrum disorder (ASD) is characterized by communication and social deficits as well as the presence of restricted and stereotypic patterns of behaviors (1). Over the past decade, estimates of the incidence of ASD have increased steadily, with a recent study finding that 60 to 66 per 10,000 are affected (2,3).

Treatment of ASD includes a range of empirically-based psychosocial interventions as well as pharmacological treatment. The latter have tended to focus upon addressing secondary symptoms of ASD, including attentional deficits, hyperactivity, aggressive behavior, irritability, ritualistic behaviors, self-injury, and anxiety (4).

In fact, risperidone was recently shown to be effective in treating symptoms of irritability and agitation in children with ASD (5) while other studies have shown drugs such as methylphenidate and atomoxetine to be effective in controlling overactivity and inattention (6,7). However, over the last decade a number of studies have attempted to identify possible pharmacologic treatments to address some of the core features of ASD (e.g., social and communication deficits), but with minimal success. For example, initial case reports suggested that secretin might improve communication and social functioning of children with ASD, but subsequent controlled trials found the compound to be no more effective than placebo (8). A recent controlled, multicenter trial involving the use of oral human immunoglobulin to treat GI symptoms and associated core features of ASD similarly failed to find any difference between active treatment and placebo (9).

The desire to ameliorate core deficits in ASD has led to increased interest in the use of cholinesterase inhibitors as a possible treatment option. Cholinergic afferent neurons innervate the cerebral cortex during the most dynamic periods of neuronal differentiation and synapse formation, suggesting that the cholinergic system plays a regulatory role in these events.

Experiments in rats have shown that disruption of cholinergic innervation during early postnatal development results in delayed cortical neuronal development with permanent alterations in cortical architecture and cognitive functioning (10).

Pathological abnormalities in basal forebrain (septal) cholinergic neurons have been reported in ASD, such as larger than normal size and numbers in children and smaller size and numbers in adults (11). Neurochemical abnormalities have also been observed in the cholinergic system in ASD.

These include decreased cortical M_1 receptor in the parietal cortex, decreased nicotinic receptors in the parietal and frontal cortices, and decreased $alpha_4$ and $beta_2$ nicotinic receptor subunits in the parietal cortex (12). In addition, Lee et al. (13) examined autopsy tissue from a group of individuals with ASD and intellectual disability (ID). In comparison to normal controls and non-ASD individuals with ID, the ASD group was found to have significantly greater cerebellar nicotinic alpha-4 receptor loss (which implicates abnormalities in the cholinergic neurotransmitter system). These observations suggest that cholinesterase inhibitors such as donepezil, rivastigmine and galantamine may have the potential to target the cognitive and behavioral abnormalities observed in ASD.

A few small studies have found that cholinesterase inhibitors may enhance behavioral and/or cognitive functioning among individuals with ASD. Hardan and Handen (14) conducted a retrospective study of 8 children (ages 7-19 years) with autism who had been prescribed donepezil (mean dose 9.37 mg/day). Four children were found to be responders. Significant reductions on the Irritability and Hyperactivity subscales of the Aberrant Behavior Checklist were reported. Two subjects experienced mild, transient side effects, including vomiting and increased irritability.

In the only controlled trial to date, Chez et al (15) reported significant improvement in receptive and expressive language skills as well as improvement on measures of the core features of autism (CARS: Childhood Autism Rating Scale) in a group of 43 children (ages 2-10 years) with autism or pervasive developmental disorder (PDD). The 6-week double-blind trial (utilizing a 2.5 mg/day dose) was followed by a 6-week open label trial (2.5 mg/day dose). However, the results remain difficult to interpret because between groups statistical analyses were not conducted.

In fact, on some measures the placebo group evidenced greater gains than children on active medication (16). There have also been a small number of studies of other cholinesterase inhibitors among children with autism. For example, Chez et al. (17) conducted an open label trial of rivastigmine with a group of 32 children with ASD (dose of 0.8 mg twice daily). Gains were noted in expressive language, core features of autism (based upon the Child Autism Rating Scale), as well as behavior (based upon the Conners Parent Rating Scale). There have also been three studies involving the use of galantamine (which is both an acetylcholinesterase inhibitor and nicotinic receptor modulator). Niederhofer et al. (18) conducted a double-blind, placebo-controlled crossover trial of galantamine with 20 children with ASD.

Slightly lower (but statistically significant) ratings were noted on combined parent and teacher measures of hyperactivity, irritability, poor eye contact, and inappropriate speech for galantamine in comparison to placebo. Hertzman (19) described the use of this agent in a case study of three adults with ASD (with doses ranging from 4-16 mg/day). Some improvement was noted in verbalizations and socially appropriate behavior. However, one subject discontinued treatment after developing a macular rash.

Finally, Nicolson, Craven-Thuss, and Smith (20) conducted a 12-week open label trial of galantamine (doses ranging from 12-24 mg/day) in a group of 13 children with ASD (4-17 years of age). Eight subjects were found to be responders, which included improvement on measures of irritability and social withdrawal (based upon a parent-completed Aberrant Behavior Checklist), inattention (based upon the Conners Parent Rating Scale), and anger (based upon a physician-completed Children's Psychiatric Rating Scale). However, two subjects withdrew from the trial due to a worsening of symptoms and one withdrew due to headaches.

The present double-blind, placebo-controlled trial assessed the tolerability, safety and efficacy of donepezil on cognitive and behavioral functioning in a group of children and adolescents with ASD.

It was hypothesized that donepezil would be superior to placebo for improving performance on executive functioning tasks and that such gains would be associated with similar improvement on behavioral measures and the core features of ASD. The current paper focuses upon the behavioral outcome measures of this study. The effects of donepezil on measures of executive functioning and learning has been published in a separate manuscript.

Our study

Thirty-four children and adolescents between 8 and 17 years of age with IQs of 75 and above served as subjects. All subjects met research diagnostic criteria for ASD (autistic disorder, PDD NOS, Asperger's Disorder) based upon both the Autism Diagnostic Interview – Revised (21) and the Autism Diagnostic Observation Schedule (22). Subjects prescribed concomitant psychotropic medications prior to starting the trial needed to have their dose levels maintained during study participation. Finally, subjects had to score at least 1 SD below mean (for gender and age) on either the Card Sorting Test, Verbal Fluency, or 20 Questions Test of the Delis-Kaplan Battery of Executive Function System (23). The following assessment tools were used to establish study eligibility criteria:

- *The Autism Diagnostic Interview–Revised (ADI-R)(21):* The ADI–R is a highly-structured method of eliciting information from a parent to confirm a clinical impression of ASD in children and adults. This interview tool has demonstrated excellent reliability and validity for the diagnosis of autism. The training for the ADI involves a set of didactic sessions, supervised administration by an expert interviewer, and demonstration of 90% reliability.
- *Autism Diagnostic Observation Schedule (ADOS) (22)* is an investigator-based procedure that places the child in naturalistic social situations demanding specific social and communication reactions. Although the protocol follows standard administration, the situations themselves are unstructured. Thus, the ADOS provides a sample of the child's behavior in a naturalistic setting. Behaviors are coded in the areas of social communication, social relatedness, play and imagination, and repetitive behaviors. The ADOS provides an algorithm for the diagnosis of autism, non-autistic PDD, and non-PDD.
- *WAISI (24):* The WAISI is a 4-sub-test screening tool that assesses both verbal and nonverbal functioning. It **is a reliable,** nationally standardized measure of intelligence that provides Verbal, Performance, Full Scale IQ scores. It is linked to the more comprehensive intelligence scales, the Wechsler Intelligence Scale for Children and the Wechsler Adult Intelligence Scale. The WAISI is normed for individuals from 6-0 to 80-0 years of age and has excellent reliability and validity.
- *The Diagnostic Interview for Children and Adolescents-Revised (DICA-IV)(25):* The DICA-IV was used to assess for comorbidity. The DICA-IV is a DSM-based diagnostic interview that has repeatedly been revised to reflect changes in the DSM classification system. The tool was developed for children and adolescents ages 6 to 17 and includes a computerized parent interview version. The DICA-IV provides information about onset, duration and severity of 185 symptoms.
- *Medical:* Parents provided a medical history and subjects were given a brief physical (including Tanner staging). A baseline EKG, hematology (CBC and differential; platelet count), urinalysis (urinalysis, R and M), and chemistry (albumin, astra 7, bilirubin-total, calcium, cholesterol, protein profile, SGOT, TSH, T_4) were obtained. These studies were repeated at weeks 5 and 10. Karyotyping for Fragile X syndrome was performed for subjects who had not previously been assessed.

The study was conducted across a 10-week period involving a double-blind, placebo-controlled, parallel groups design. Following a one-week baseline, subjects were randomly assigned to either active medication or placebo. The study pharmacist conducted the randomization for each subject based upon tanner stage (stages 1-2 versus 3-5) and gender. Subjects began at a 2.5 mg/day dose, which was increased to 5.0 mg/day after a week. Following a total of four weeks at 5.0 mg/day, subjects were re-evaluated. They subsequently had their doses increased to 7.5 mg/day for a one-week period, following by a final titration to 10.0 mg/day for the remaining four weeks of the trial. Subjects returned to the clinic for a cognitive re-assessment following a total of four weeks on 10.0 mg/day.

Following randomization, subjects were seen for a total of 4 clinic visits (following one week on 2.5 mg/day, four weeks on 5 mg/day, one week at 7.5 mg/day, and four weeks at 10 mg/day). The visits at weeks 1 and 6 were only conducted to assess safety and to determine if the subject would be able to have his/her medication titrated to the next dose level. If side effects developed and were interfering with a subject's functioning or well-being, the dose was reduced to previous the highest dose and maintained at that level for the duration of the study. In cases where problems persisted, the subject was brought to the clinic for a final assessment and the medication discontinued.

Families were encouraged to contact study staff should the subject experience any concerning side effects. Families were contacted via telephone at least once between study visits. Compliance was assessed by having families complete a daily log, tracking when medication was given and noting if there were any problems. The use of concomitant medications (e.g., aspirin, cold medicine) was also noted in the log. Families returned the medication dispenser at each visit for a pill count.

Medication was packed by the hospital research pharmacy, with both active medication and placebo placed in opaque capsules. At the conclusion of the double-blind trial, subjects who had been assigned to placebo were offered a 10-week open-label trial (utilizing the identical titration schedule). Open-label subjects were re-assessed at week 5 (5 mg/day dose) and week 10 (10 mg/day dose). The following dependent measures were obtained at baseline, week 5, and week 10 for behavioral functioning:

- *The Clinical Global Impression Scale (CGIS) (26).* This clinician rating scale consists of 3 subscales: severity of illness, global improvement, and therapeutic index. The severity of the illness is scored from 1= normal to 7= extremely ill. The patient's improvement is scored in a 7-point scale which ranges from marked improved (1), to no change (4), and to very much worse (7). The CGIS has been widely use in psychopharmacological studies and has been shown to be highly sensitive to medication effects. Consistent with the Autism RUPP Network (27), a score of 3 (mildly ill) on the severity of illness scale was assigned to subjects based upon the core features of ASD. Higher scores were assigned based upon the presence of other, secondary behaviors. The scores on the severity of illness and improvement scale were based upon parent interview, parent-completed behavior problem checklists, as well as direct observation of the subject. The scale was completed by a study team member who was not involved in assessing side effects or controlling drug dosing.
- *Child Behavior Checklist (CBCL):* The CBCL (28) was used to assess behavioral issues. The CBCL is a well standardized, broad-band rating scale that has been

widely used in research and for clinical purposes to assess the presence of behavioral and emotional problems in school-aged children. The 118 items comprise nine subscales: 1) withdrawn; 2) somatic complaints; 3) anxious / depressed; 4) social problems; 5) thought problems 6) attention problems; 7) delinquent problems; 8) aggressive behavior; 9) sex problems. In addition to the nine subscale scores, a total problem score and two broad-band scores (internalizing and externalizing) may be calculated.

- *The Real Life Rating Scale (RLRS)(29):* A modified version of the RLRS was completed by parents at baseline and weeks 5 and 10. The RLRS is designed to measure behavior in children with ASD over time and across treatments. A total of 47 behaviors in five categories are coded: Sensory Motor (e.g., hand flapping, rocking), Social Relationship to People (e.g., appropriate responses to interaction attempts), Affectual Responses (e.g., crying, temper outbursts), Sensory Responses (e.g., sniffing self or others), and Language (e.g., communicative use of language). In addition, there is a total score. Items were rated using a 4-point scale: 0 ("never"), 1 ("infrequently"), 2 ("frequently"), 3 ("almost always"). Ratings of normal behaviors are subtracted from three of the five scales, which could result in negative values in some cases. The RLRS served as a primary measure with which to assess global changes in the core features of ASD. The RLRS was used as a parent questionnaire (rather than as a direct observation system) most recently by the Research Units on Pediatric Psychopharmacology to document the effects of risperidone on restricted, repetitive and stereotyped patterns of behavior. However, no gains on social interactions or communication were found (30).

Statistical analysis

Data were analyzed by using statistical software, SPSS® (SPSS inc. Chicago, IL) version 15 with general linear model (GLM) repeated measures procedures to run a repeated measures analysis of variance (ANOVA).

For double-blinded data, one between group factor and one within subject factor studies were used. The between group factor was the drug conditions (drug and placebo) and the within subjects factor was the time (baseline, 5 mg dose in week 5, and 10 mg dose in week 10). For open-label data, within-subject studies were used. A test of sphericity assumption was performed. If the assumption was violated, corrections (either Greenhouse-Geisser or Huynh-Feldt) were made to the F test. Where appropriate, post-hoc tests were conducted. Bonferroni adjustment test was used for pairwise comparisons. For subjects who did not complete the entire 10-week protocol due to the appearance of significant adverse side effects, an intent-to-treatment approach was employed by the last observation being carried forward (LOCF). Any final observations during the active treatment or placebo phase that was conducted prior to the end of the trial were carried forward as if they had occurred at the 5 or 10-week mark. If there were no statistically significant different conclusions between the repeated measures ANOVA above and the LOCF repeated measures ANOVA, the latter were used. For the open label donepezil trial (for placebo non-responders), a repeated measures ANOVA was similarly used with LOCF for subjects who were unable to complete the trial.

Our findings

Thirty-four subjects were randomized for the trial and 31 were able to complete the entire protocol as designed. One subject terminated due to an increase in aggression and irritability. Two other subjects were unable to tolerate the 10 mg/day dose and were maintained on a 5 mg/day dose. No statistially significant differences between groups were found for age, gender, IQ or ADOS score.

Mean age for the active medication group was 8 years 7 months while the mean age for the placebo group was 9 years 7 months.

Mean full scale IQ scores were 96.8 and 96.7, respectively; mean severity of autism symptoms (as measured by the Total score on the ADOS) was 10.2 and 11.2, respectively. Eleven subjects were prescribed a single concomitant medication prior to entering the trial. Of these, five subjects were prescribed SSRIs, four were prescribed stimulants, and two were prescribed atomoxetine.

Table 1 summarizes the results of the CGI and CBCL subscales at baseline, 5 mg, and 10 mg/day doses. While decreases on most subscales were noted during both drug doses in comparison to baseline, no statistically significant differences between active medication and placebo were found on the between group analyses.

The CBCL Total Problems decreased significantly for both treatment groups, from a mean of 60.1 to 51.9 for those on active medication and from a mean of 60.1 to 46.1 for those on placebo.

The between group analysis was not significant. Parents also reported statistically significant decreases on sub-scales such as Thought Problems, Social Problems and Aggression for both groups. But again, no statistically significant between group differences were found. Similar findings were noted for the CGI, where only minimal ratings of improvement were noted for subjects.

Table 2 summarizes the results of the Ritvo Freeman (RLRS). As with the CBCL, no significant between group differences were noted. Significant improvement (indicated by a lower score) on a number of the Ritvo-Freeman subscales assessing the core features of ASD were found.

These occurred only during the 5 mg dose for Sensory Motor (placebo only), Social Relationships (for both conditions), Sensory Responses (placebo only), and Total Score (both conditions).

However, none of the between group post-hoc analyses were found to be statistically significant.

Tables 3 and 4 provide the results of the open label donepezil trial for 14 subjects who had been assigned placebo. On the CBCL, no statistically significant differences between baseline and the 5 mg dose, between baseline and the 10 mg dose, or between the 5 mg and 10 mg dose were noted (see Table 3).

For core features of autism (Ritvo-Freeman), improvements were noted at the 5 mg dose and remained fairly stable at the 10 mg dose. However, no gains were found to be statistically significant (see Table 4).

Table 1. Double-blind trial: CBCL raw score means and standard deviations

Dependent Measures	Baseline		5 mg		10 mg		Between Groups p
	Drug	Placebo	Drug	Placebo	Drug	Placebo	
Anxiety	7.78 (4.89)	9.33 (5.85)	7.17 (4.27)	7.80 (5.87)[1]	7.44 (4.41)	8.07 (5.24)	0.579
Withdrawn	5.06 (3.19)	6.73 (2.71)	4.28 (2.76)	5.53 (2.80)[1]	4.44 (2.81)	5.93 (3.15)	0.111
Somatic Complaints	2.00 (2.85)	1.73 (2.96)	1.83 (2.01)	1.67 (3.60)	1.72 (1.84)	1.13 (1.89)	0.690
Social Problems	7.44 (4.88)	8.00 (5.40)	6.17 (4.15)[1]	6.67 (4.75)	6.17 (4.03)	5.73 (4.57)[2]	0.893
Thought Problems	7.17 (2.83)	7.73 (3.86)	5.67 (2.70)[1]	6.60 (4.14)	5.00 (2.33)[3]	5.60 (3.48)[2]	0.498
Attention	11.56 (4.00)	11.13 (3.72)	10.56 (3.58)[1]	9.27 (3.94)[3]	10.61 (4.10)	8.67 (4.08)[3]	0.353
Rule Break	2.94 (1.80)	2.67 (2.77)	2.33 (2.06)	2.00 (2.65)	1.94 (1.73)[1]	1.87 (2.50)	0.747
Aggression	9.72 (6.09)	7.47 (5.72)	7.83 (6.24)[1]	5.67 (4.44)[1]	8.39 (6.28)	5.20 (3.14)[1]	0.170
Affect Total	5.00(3.68)	6.40 (4.12)	3.72 (2.65)[1]	4.40 (3.38)[2]	4.00 (2.70)	4.33 (2.97)[1]	0.433
Anxiety Total	5.00 (3.05)	5.20 (3.30)	4.44 (2.73)	4.33 (3.27)[1]	4.39 (3.01)	4.53 (3.11)	0.939
Somatic Total	1.06 (1.92)	0.73 (1.58)	0.89 (1.32)	0.87 (2.17)	0.61 (0.92)	0.67 (1.23)	0.850
ADHD Total	8.33 (3.58)	6.93 (3.24)	8.06 (3.52)	5.80 (3.08)[1]	7.67 (3.43)	5.07 (2.82)[3]	0.064
ODD Total	3.89 (2.61)	3.53 (2.70)	3.17 (2.46)	2.73 (2.12)	3.61 (2.72)	2.53 (1.64)	0.408
CD Total	3.83 (2.73)	3.33 (4.15)	2.50 (2.26)[2]	2.13 (3.42)[1]	2.89 (2.78)[1]	2.27 (3.58)[1]	0.638
Internal Total	14.83 (8.69)	17.80 (8.62)	13.28 (7.24)	15.00 (8.92)[1]	13.61 (7.34)	15.13 (8.21)	0.443
External Total	12.67 (6.92)	10.13 (7.63)	10.17 (7.66)[1]	7.67 (6.07)[1]	10.33 (7.53)[1]	7.07 (4.98)[1]	0.229
Total Problem	60.11 (21.37)	60.13 (20.60)	52.17 (21.39)[2]	50.20 (21.49)[2]	51.89 (22.85)[1]	46.13 (18.83)[3]	0.713

[1]=p<.05; [2]=p<.01; [3]=p<.001.

Table 2. Double–blind trial: Other behavioral means and standard deviations

Dependent Measures	Baseline		5 mg		10 mg		Between Groups p
	Drug	Placebo	Drug	Placebo	Drug	Placebo	
CGI-Imp	-	-	3.56 (0.62)	3.60 (0.63)	3.50 (0.86)	3.47 (0.64)	.979
CGI-Sev	3.88 (0.60)	3.93 (0.59)	3.65 (0.49)	3.73 (0.46)	3.65 (0.70)	3.67 (0.62)	.770
RLRS (raw score means)							
Sensory Motor	.46 (.41)	.45 (.54)	.39 (.47)	.33 (.42)[1]	.46 (.45)	.42 (.48)	.823
Social Relationships	.26 (.36)	.34 (.55)	-.001 (.40)[2]	.003 (.46)[3]	.15 (.45)	.17 (.49)	.798
Affectual Responses	.90 (.55)	.80 (.68)	.86 (.67)	.65 (.46)	.94 (.67)	.67 (.59)	.310
Sensory Responses	.63 (.46)	.59 (.45)	.51 (.51)	.41 (.50)[1]	.56 (.56)	.50 (.45)	.676
Language	-.09 (.34)	-.09 (.39)	-.20 (.37)	-.20 (.45)	-.18 (.36)	-.17 (.44)	.976
Total Score	.43 (.30)	.42 (.38)	.31 (.39)[1]	.24 (.34)[2]	.39 (.37)	.32 (.39)	.665

[1]=$p<.05$; [2]=$p<.01$; [3]=$p<.001$

Table 3. Open label trial: CBCL raw score means and standard deviations

	Baseline*	5 mg	10 mg	Baseline vs 5 mg	Baseline vs 10 mg	5 mg vs 10 mg
Anxiety	8.23 (5.09)	8.08 (5.11)	7.77 (5.21)	P=.999	P=.999	P=.999
Withdrawn	6.00 (3.24)	5.92 (2.72)	6.00 (2.68)	P=.999	P=.999	P=.999
Somatic Complaints	0.69 (1.03)	0.62 (0.96)	0.62 (.096)	P=.999	P=.999	P=.999
Social Problems	6.08 (4.80)	6.38 (4.79)	6.31 (3.91)	P=.999	P=.999	P=.999
Thought Problems	5.31 (3.38)	5.31 (3.33)	5.85 (4.30)	P=.999	P=.999	P=.999
Attention	8.85 (4.34)	8.69 (4.52)	8.46 (4.27)	P=.999	P=.999	P=.999
Rule Break	2.15 (2.58)	2.69 (2.75)	2.38 (3.01)	P=.838	P=.999	P=.999
Aggression	5.92 (2.69)	5.77 (5.36)	5.62 (4.35)	P=.999	P=.999	P=.999
Affect Total	4.15 (2.82)	4.38 (2.99)	4.77 (2.95)	P=.999	P=.999	P=.999
Anxiety Total	4.92 (3.07)	4.54 (2.85)	4.15 (3.02)	P=.999	P=.741	P=.999
Somatic Total	0.38 (0.87)	0.23 (0.60)	0.08 (0.28)	P=.999	P=.312	P=.496
ADHD Total	5.15 (2.97)	5.46 (3.04)	4.77 (3.09)	P=.999	P=.999	P=.632
ODD Total	2.85 (1.52)	2.85 (2.54)	2.69 (1.80)	P=.999	P=.999	P=.999
CD Total	2.62 (3.73)	2.85 (3.83)	2.85 (3.76)	P=.999	P=.999	P=.999
Internal Total	14.92 (7.50)	14.62 (7.21)	14.38 (6.46)	P=.999	P=.999	P=.999
External Total	8.08 (4.54)	8.46 (7.21)	8.00 (5.89)	P=.999	P=.999	P=.999
Total Problem	47.38 (19.07)	47.69 (25.23)	47.23 (21.14)	P=.999	P=.999	P=.999

*baseline is the results of the final visit of the double-blind trial .

Table 4. Open label trial: Other behavioral means and standard deviations

Dependent Measures	Baseline	5 mg	10 mg	Baseline vs 5 mg	Baseline vs 10 mg	5 mg vs 10 mg
CGI- Imp.	3.54 (0.52)	3.62 (0.51)	3.69 (0.48)	P=.999	P=.900	P=.999
CGI-Sev	3.77 (0.60)	3.63 (0.51)	3.69 (0.48)	P=.999	P=.900	P=.999
RLRS (raw score means)						
Sensory Motor	.44 (.51)	.28 (.40)	.29 (.48)	P=.338	P=.192	P=.999
Social Relationships	.26 (.51)	.14 (.47)	.14 (.51)	P=.649	P=.513	P=.999
Affectual Responses	.73 (.61)	.62 (.56)	.69 (.54)	P=.999	P=.900	P=.999
Sensory Responses	.53 (.49)	.35 (.35)	.35 (.40)	P=.060	P=.106	P=.999
Language	-.08 (.42)	-.24 (.38)	-.38 (.38)	P=.325	P=.019	P=.213
Total Score	.39 (.41)	.23 (.33)	.22 (.37)	P=.119	P=.079	P=.999

Discussion

This paper presents the results of the behavioral measures from a double-blind, placebo-controlled trial of donepezil in 34 children and adolescents with ASD. The findings are consistent with a number of other recent medication trials in the autism field in which there was a high rate of placebo response and no significant differences noted between the two treatment groups (9, 31). Subjects tended to improve for both conditons with scores either stabalizing or lessening slightly in affect during the second (10 mg) assessment. The most significant finding is that this study differs considerably from prior research studies in this area, where postive results were noted (14, 15). One possible explanation for the difference between the current study outcome and that of Chez et al (15) is that the latter study used a much younger age group (but also a lower medication dose). It may be that the effects of cognitive enhancers, such as donepezil, are limited to children who are still in their earlier stages of development. Also as discussed earlier the Chez et al study failed to conduct between group analyses (only reporting within group statistics). Therefore, it is somewhat difficult to compar the results of these two studies.

The current study findings also differ from our own initial open label study where subjects were found to have significant decreases on the Irritability and Hyperactivity subscales of the Aberrant Behavior Checklist (14). However, the subjects in our open trial were prescribed donepezil due to high baseline ratings on the Conners (and were also on a number of concomitant medications). This type of behavioral inclusion was not requried for the randomized trial. Yet, when donepezil was put to the test in a double-blind manner, both the placebo and active medication groups reported improvement. In fact, as a group, those on placebo tended to fare better (demonstrating statistically significant gains on a total of 24 comparisions vs 15 comparisons for the active medication group). In addition, p levels for the placebo group also tended to be higher (10 out of 24 with a $p \leq .01$ or $p \leq .001$ for placebo versus 4 out of 15 for the active medication group). Such results would suggest that the findings on prior open label studies were likely placebo responses.

Despite being a well-controlled study, there are a number of methodological issues that may have impacted the final outcome. First, subjects were selected based primarily upon a diagnosis of ASD. Significant behavioral deficits were not an inclusion criteria. Consequently, there may have been relatively limited range for improvement on many of the measures. It is also possible that there were subjects who experienced gains that we were not able to capture with the scales selected for use in the study. Another explanation for the lack of significant treatment effects is that a longer period of time is required to impact a subject's behavior and/or the core features of ASD. Ten weeks may simply have not provided enough time to detect improvement in these areas. The most striking finding of this study was the robust placebo affect reported by parents across the 10-week period. In addition, the fact that subjects on open-label donepezil at the end of the double-blind study continued to evidence some gains makes interpretation of the findings difficult.

Additional controlled trials that include long-term follow-up of the use of cholinesterase inhibitors in this population may be needed. Other cognitive enahancers, such as memantine (a NMDA receptor antagonist), may have a greater impact on the behavior of children and adolescents with ASD. Future studies should also include younger children as well as individuals with significant ASD symptoms. Inclusion criteria should specify specific behavioral and cognitive deficits as well. This current study provides further evidence of the importance of conducting carefully controlled, double-blind psychopharmacological studies in the ASD field and reminds clinicians that this is the only way to develop evidence-based treatment guidelines for this challenging population.

Acknowledgments

This study was supported by NIMH grant #5R21 MH64941-03 (Treating Cognitive Deficits in Autism) as well as by a gift by Pfizer and Eisai Pharmaceutical Companies (who also provided the medication and placebo for this trial). We wish to acknowledge Janine Janosky, Ph.D. and Qing Sun, Ph.D. for their assistance in conducting the statistical analysis for this project as well as Patricia Joe Murray, Ph.D., for conducting the neuropsychological assessments. We also thank all of the subjects and their families who participated in this study.

References

[1] American Psychiatric Association. Diagnostic and statistical manual of mental disorders, 5th ed. Washington, DC: Am. Psychiatr. Assoc., 2000.

[2] CDC. Prevalence of autism spectrum disorders--autism and developmental disabilities monitoring network, 14 sites, United States, 2002, MMWR 2007;56:12-28.

[3] Fombonne E. Epidemiology of autistic disorder and other pervasive developmental disorders. J. Clin. Psychiatr. 2005;10:3-8.

[4] Handen BL, Lubetsky MJ. Psychopharmacology in autism. Sch. Psychol. Quart. 2005;20:155-71.

[5] McCracken JT, McGough J, Shah B, Cronin P, Hong D, Aman MG, et al. Risperidone in children with autism and serious behavioral problems. New. Engl. J. Med. 2002;347;314–21.

[6] Arnold LE. Aman MG. Cook AM. Witwer AN. Hall KL. Thompson S. Ramadan Y. Atomoxetine for hyperactivity in autism spectrum disorders: placebo-controlled crossover pilot trial. J. Am. Acad. Child Adolesc. Psychiatr. 2006;45:1196-1205.

[7] Research Units on Pediatric Psychopharmacology Autism Network. A randomized, double-blind, placebo-controlled, crossover trial of methylphenidate in children with hyperactivity associated with pervasive developmental disorders. Arch. Gen. Psychiatr. 2005;62:1266–74.

[8] Sturmey P. Secretin is an ineffective treatment for pervasive developmental disabilities: a review of 15 double-blind randomized controlled trials Res. Dev. Disabil. 2005;26:87-97.

[9] Handen, BL Melmed RD, Hansen RL, Aman MG, Burnham D, Bruss J, McDougle CJ. A double-blind, placebo-controlled trial of oral human immunoglobulin for gastrointestinal dysfunction in children with autistic disorder. J. Autism Dev. Disord. 2009;39:796-805.

[10] Hohmann C, Berger-Sweeney J. Cholinergic regulation of cortical development and plasticity: New twists to an old story. Perspect. Dev. Neurobiol. 1998;5:401-25.

[11] Bauman ML, Kemper TL. Neuroanatomic observations of the brain in autism. In: Bauman M , Kemper T. The neurobiology of autism. Baltimore, MD: Johns Hopkins Univ. Press, 1994:119-45.

[12] Perry E, Lee M, Martin-Ruiz C, Court J, Volsen S, Merrit J, et al. Cholinergic activity in autism: Abnormalities in the cerebral cortex and basal forebrain. Am. J. Psychiatr. 2001;158:1058-66.

[13] Lee M, Martin-Ruiz C, Graham A, Court J, Jaros E, Perry R, et al. Nicotinic receptor abnormalities in the cerebellar cortex in autism Brain 2002;125:1482-95.

[14] Hardan AY, Handen BL. A retrospective open trial of adjunctive donepezil in children and adolescents with autistic disorder. J. Child Adolesc. Psychopharmacol. 2002;12:237-41.

[15] Chez MG, Buchanan TM, Becker M, Kessler J, Aimonovitch MC, Mrazek SR. Donepezil hydrochloride: A double-blind study in autistic children. J. Pediatr. Neurol. 2003;1:83–8.
[16] Yoo HJ, Valdovinos HG, Williams DC. Relevance of donepezil in enhancing learning and memory in special populations: A Review of the Literature. J. Autism Dev. Disord. 2007;37:1883-901.
[17] Chez MG, Aimonovitch M, Buchanan T, Mrazek S, Tremb RJ. Treating autistic spectrum disorders in children: utility of the cholinesterase inhibitor rivastigmine tartrate. J. Child Neurol. 2004;19:165-69.
[18] Niederhofer H, Staffen W, Mair A. Galantamine may be effective in treating autistic disorder. Br. J. Med. 2002;325:1422.
[19] Hertzman M. Galantamine in the treatment of adult autism: A report of three clinical cases. Int. J. Psychiatr. Med. 2003;33:395-98.
[20] Nicholson R, Craven-Thuss B, Smith JJ. A prospective, open-label trial of galantamine in autistic disorder. J. Child Adolesc. Psychopharmacol. 2006;16:621-29.
[21] Rutter M, Le Couteur A, Lord C. Autism diagnostic interview-revised. Los Angeles, CA: Western Psychol. Serv., 2003.
[22] Lord C, Rutter M, DiLavore PC, Risi S. Autism diagnostic observation schedule: A standardized observation of communicative and social behavior. Los Angeles, CA: Western Psychol. Serv., 1999.
[23] Delis C, Kaplan E, Kramer JH. Delis-Kaplan Executive function system: Technical manual. San Antonio, TX: Psychol. Corp., 2001.
[24] Wechsler D. Wechsler Abbreviated Scale of Intelligence. San San Antonio, TX: Psychol. Corp., 1999.
[25] Reich W, Welner Z, Herjanic B, and the MHS Staff. Manual for the diagnostic interview for children and adolescents-IV (DICA-IV). North Tonawanda, NY: Multi-Health System, 1997.
[26] Guy W. ECDEU Assessment Manual of Psychopharmacology. Rockville, MD.: Natl. Inst. Mental Health, 1976;76-338.
[27] Arnold LE, Aman MG, Martin A, Collier-Crespin A, Vitiello B, Tierney E, et al. Assessment in multisite randomized clinical trials (RCTs) of patients with autistic disorder. J. Autism Dev. Disord. 2000;30:99-111.
[28] Achenbach TM. Manual for ASEBA School-Age Form. Burlington VT: Univ Vermont, Res Center Youth Fam., 2001.
[29] Freeman BJ, Ritvo ER, Yokota A, Ritvo A. A scale for rating symptoms of patients with the syndrome of autism in real life settings. J. Am. Acad. Child Adol. Psychiatry 1986;25:130-36.
[30] McDougle CJ, Scahill L, Aman MG, McCracken J, Tierney E, Davies M, et al. Risperidone for the core symptom domains of Autism: Results from the study by the Autism Network of the Research Units on Pediatric Psychopharmacology. Am. J. Psychiatr. 2005;162:1142-48.
[31] King BH. Hollander E. Sikich L. McCracken JT. Scahill L. Bregman JD, et al. Lack of efficacy of citalopram in children with autism spectrum disorders and high levels of repetitive behavior: citalopram ineffective in children with autism Arch. Gen. Psychiatr. 2009;66:583-90.

In: Understanding Autism Spectrum Disorder
Editors: Ditza A Zachor and Joav Merrick
ISBN: 978-1-62081-353-9

Chapter 12

Abnormal white matter in language-related brain tracts in non-verbal children with autism

Yonata Levy[1,2], **Dafna Ben Bashat**[3], **Liat Ben Sira**[3], **Talma Hendler**[3,4], **Esther Ben Itzchak**[6,7], **Vered Kronfeld-Duenias**[3,5] **and Ditza A. Zachor**[4,6]*

[1]Department of Psychology, Hebrew University, Jerusalem, Israel
[2]Hadassah-Hebrew University Medical School, Jerusalem, Israel
[3]Wohl Institute for Advanced Imaging, Functional Brain Imaging Center, Tel Aviv Sourasky Medical Center, Tel Aviv, Israel
[4]Sackler Faculty of Medicine, Tel Aviv University, Tel Aviv
[5]Lester and Sally Entin Faculty of Humanities, Tel Aviv University, Tel Aviv, Israel
[6]Department of Pediatrics, Autism Center, Assaf Harofeh Medical Center, Zerifin, Israel
[7]Department of Communication Disorders, Ariel University Center, Ariel, Israel

Abstract

Children with autism spectrum disorder (ASD) show great variability in their language abilities. The current longitudinal study examined brain white matter maturation in four toddlers with autism, mean age 2.3 years, who were pre-verbal at the time of diagnosis. After one year of intensive intervention the children were re-evaluated, for their autism status as well as for language and cognitive levels. The second evaluation confirmed the diagnosis of autism. It also established the fact that two children were non-verbal, while the other two developed complex language. Imaging results showed abnormal integrity in

* Correspondence: Professor Yonata Levy, PhD, Department of Psychology, Hebrew University, Mount Scopus IL-91905 Jerusalem, Israel. E-mail: msyonata@huji.ac.il

overall analysis and in selected regions of interest in all four children. High b value DWI revealed abnormal diffusivities values and increased anisotropy in the left- superior longitudinal fasciculus, which is a fiber tract connecting Broca's and Wernicke's areas, solely in the non-verbal children. It is proposed that abnormal white matter integrity in language-related tracts may correlate with language development in autism.

Introduction

Children with autism spectrum disorder (ASD) show great variability with respect to language performance (1). About 25-40% of the individuals with autism are 'non-verbal' or mute with figures depending largely on the definition of 'non-verbal' (2). Structural and fMRI studies of language-related areas in children and adults with ASD suggested deviations from normal. Wilcox et al (3) found age related changes in hypoperfusion of verbal-associated left-temporal lobe and frontal areas in children with autism.

These changes correlated with language development and with cognitive performance during maturation. Herbert et al (4) reported reversed right-left cerebral cortex asymmetry ratio in individuals with autism, confined to smaller units of the cerebral cortex. Flagg et al (5) found that children with autism followed opposite maturational trajectories in language lateralization to those observed in typically developing (TD) children. De Fosse et al (6) reported of reversed asymmetry patterns between left and right frontal regions in participants with autism who were language impaired. Similar reversed asymmetries were seen in participants with specific language impairment (SLI), yet not in participants with autism who had normal language. Reported volumes of these regions suggested that the asymmetry stemmed from decreased left hemisphere volume, as well as increased right hemisphere volume, in the two language-impaired populations. Redcay and Courchesne (7) found delayed and deviant patterns of brain responses to speech presented during sleep in a group of ten 3 year old children with ASD.

Diffusion tensor imaging (DTI) and the related, high b value diffusion weighted imaging (DWI), have been used to study white matter integrity. DTI provides three important parameters: the first is the average extent of water diffusion, which provides information on restriction and boundaries (Apparent Diffusion Constant –ADC, i.e. the extent of the packing density of cells). ADC decreases during normal development. The second parameter concerns the degree of diffusion anisotropy that is higher in dense and ordered structures (fractional anisotropy-FA). FA increases during normal development. The third concerns the orientation of the ordered structure (8-10). While conventional MRI shows brain developmental changes mainly up to the age of two, studies of normal white matter maturation using DTI show changes in ADC and FA throughout development and into adulthood (11-12). DTI studies, investigating white matter structure in adolescence and young adults with autism, reported reduced FA and increased mean diffusivity in several brain areas (17-19).

Two additional sets of images can be extracted from high b value diffusion weighted imaging (DWI) thru the use of q-space analysis - probability (Prob) and displacement (Disp) - representing the displacement distribution function of the water molecules (13). DWI was shown to be sensitive to white matter integrity and maturation both during normal development and in various pathological processes (13-16). Ben Bashat et al (20) examined DTI and high b value DWI in very young children with autism (1.8-3.3y). Tractography analysis showed increased defusivity in the mid-body of the corpus callosum but not in the left-SLF (21). Results indicate higher anisotropy in toddlers with autism in overall white matter pixel count and in several brain regions including the left superior longitudinal fasciculus.

The current study rests on the assumption that failure to acquire language will be reflected in abnormal structural properties of white matter fiber tracts. Our view connects with the model of autism as a network disorder that is crucially affected by structural and functional deficits of interconnectivity within the brain (21, 22).It is predicted that developmental white matter abnormalities, detectable at a young age, will signal risk of failure to acquire language.

The study

Four boys ages 1.11 – 2.10 (mean age 2.3 years) were diagnosed with autism using the Autism Diagnosis Interview-Revised (ADI-R; 23) and the Autism Diagnosis Observation Schedule (ADOS;24) module 1, and based on DSM-IV criteria (25). Participants had undergone a cognitive evaluation using the Bailey Scales of Infant Development (26), and all were at a pre-verbal stage. The children were right handed and had caring families of low to moderate socio-economic status. Following initial diagnosis, a conventional MRI, DTI and high b value DWI were acquired.

Subsequently, the children were enrolled in the same early intensive behavioral-educational program and received one-on-one, 25 hours/week of intervention that focused on language, socialization, cognitive and adaptive skills. After one year of intervention, the children were re-evaluated for the status of their autism classification using the ADOS diagnostic tool (new algorithm; 27) and based on DSM-IV criteria.

Cognitive level was assessed using the Stanford Binet Intelligence Scale (28) and language abilities were re-examined. Note that the current study follows Schuler's definition of 'non-verbal' that includes individuals who produce no vocalization at all, individuals who produce only meaningless vocalizations, as well as individuals who use a limited number of words and no word combinations to express immediate desires (29). Evaluations at both times were conducted by a pediatric neurologist, and by examiners who had previously established reliability on the ADI-R and ADOS tests as required.

Control group: Forty one MR scans (18 boys) were acquired from typically developing subjects (TD), ages 4 months to 23 years (mean age: 9.6). Children up to ten years of age were referred for the following indications: febrile convulsion, intermittent torticollis, suspected endocrine abnormalities and suspected brain abnormalities on prenatal ultrasound. Only subjects without any brain anomalies on MRI as judged by a child neuro-radiologist were included in this study. Subjects ten years of age and older were recruited specifically for the current study. This group served as a control group in an earlier DTI study (20).

Additional requirements for eligibility included normal developmental history, attendance of a regular school, no history of seizures or head injury, no hearing loss. Parents or participants signed an informed consent form. The Institutional Review Board of the Tel-Aviv Sourasky Medical Center and the Israeli Ministry of Health approved the MRI and sedation protocols as detailed below.

Diagnostic tools

Autism Diagnostic Interview- Revised (ADI –R). This is a semi-structured interview administered to parents. It is designed to make a diagnosis of autism according to DSM-IV criteria (23,25). Autism Diagnosis Observation Schedule (ADOS). This is a semi-structured, interactive schedule designed to assess social and communicative functioning. The new ADOS diagnostic algorithm that classifies children into categories of autism, ASD or non-spectrum was used (24,27).

The Bayley Scales of Infant Development, 2nd Edition. This is a widely used measure of infant development that has well-developed norms and good reliability and validity. The BSID-II is administered to healthy children ages 1-42 months (26). The Stanford-Binet Intelligence Scale Fourth Edition was used with verbal children. The test measures overall cognitive development as well as four different cognitive domains – verbal reasoning, quantitative reasoning, abstract/visual reasoning, and short-term memory skills (M = 100; SD = ±15; 28).

Image acquisition

MRI was performed on a 1.5 T (GE Signa Horizon, Echo speed, LX MRI scanner, Milwaukee, WI, USA). The protocol included anatomical sequences - sagittal T_1 and axial T_2, weighted images as well as axial, FLAIR and coronal T_2 weighted images. The calculated diffusion maps were obtained from a series of 8 diffusion gradients with a maximum b value of 6,000 s/mm^2, performed at 6 non-collinear gradient directions.

Sedation protocol: When necessary, participants under the age of ten underwent light sedation with a gas mixture of nitrous oxide in 40% oxygen enriched with halothane 0.6-0.8%. Subjects breathed spontaneously through a laryngeal mask airway. EKG, pulse oximetry and capnography were monitored. Older, cooperative participants among the controls were scanned without sedation.

Data analysis

Three sets of images were extracted from high b value DTI scans- FA, Prob and Disp. FA maps were calculated from thirty-one volumes acquired at different low b values. Prob and Disp maps were obtained, using q-space analysis for the entire diffusion data set (20). Diffusivities indices were analyzed with in-house software written in Matlab©. Overall white matter pixels count (WMPC) and region of interest (ROI) analyses were performed on the three calculated indices (FA, Prob and Disp). In the first analysis, the number of pixels representing mature white matter was calculated for each subject from a histogram averaged on all acquired slices. In the second level analysis, quantitative ROI measurements were performed in 20 anatomical regions in the brain, 18 prescribed in the white matter as shown on figure 1 (A-D), and two in the gray matter. Regions of white matter were manually prescribed on color-coded DTI, segmenting the fibers according to their presumed directions. Between-judge reliability, as measured by Pearson correlation was r= 0.9. ROIs in the white matter were selected according to Mori et al (30) atlas of human white matter and prescribed separately for each hemisphere. When possible, ROIs were defined on more than one slice. White matter ROIs were: genu of the corpus callosum, splenium of the corpus callosum, anterior limb of the internal capsule, posterior limb of the internal capsule, external capsule, forceps minor and forceps major, cortico-spinal tract and the superior longitudinal fasciculus (SLF). In the gray matter, the inferior frontal gyrus (IFG, also known as Brodman areas 44-45 but including the fronto-operculus region) was defined anatomically assuming its correspondence to the functional gray matter Broca's area. Averaged values of FA, Prob and Disp were computed for each white matter ROIs. For the gray matter IFG, high b value DWI analysis showed values for Disp and Prob, yet FA values could not be obtained (20).

A mono-exponential function with least squares curve fitting (y=a1+a2*exp (-age/a3)), where y stands for FA/Prob/Disp values, was used to produce developmental curves and a predicted band of 95% was calculated.

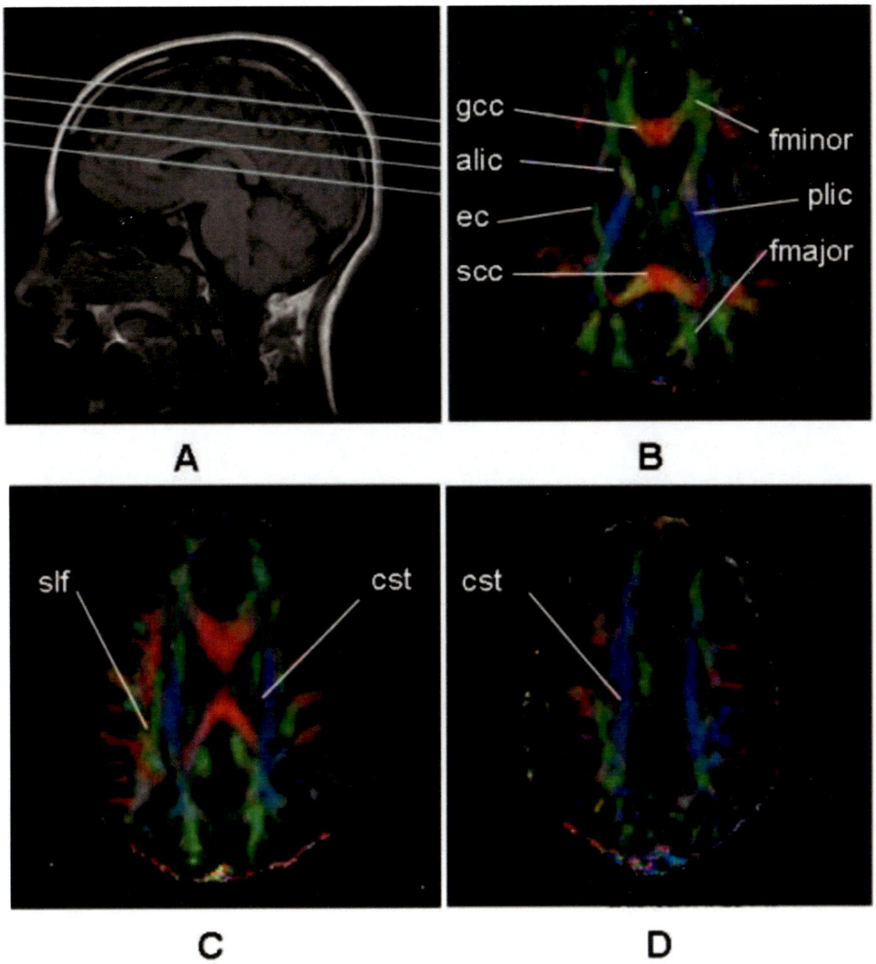

Figure 1. Sagittal image of the brain, with lines representing the location of the acquired slices (A). Selected ROIs prescribed on color coded DTI (B-D). The colors represent different directions: blue for superior–inferior, red for left–right, and green for anterior–posterior. gcc: genu of the corpus callosum; scc: splenium of the corpus callosum; alic: anterior limb of the internal capsule; plic: posterior limb of the internal capsule; ec: external capsule; fminor; forceps minor; fmajor: forceps major; slf: superior longitudinal fasciculus; cst: cortico spinal tract.

In the gray matter areas a logarithmic function with least squares curve fitting was used to produce developmental curves. Data points for child A, B, C and D were plotted against these curves.

Findings

Autism diagnosis category: All four participants acquired a diagnosis of autism disorder and reached the cutoff points for autism on the ADI and ADOS module 1 (new algorithm), at baseline Following one year of intervention, patients A and B were assessed with ADOS Module 2, which is used for children with spontaneous sentences of three or more words, while patients C and D, whose language included few spontaneous single words, were assessed on ADOS module 1. Importantly, all four children remained above the cutoff point for autism as defined by the ADOS new algorithm. Patients A and B showed improvement in autism symptoms severity in all the examined domains, whereas autism symptoms continued to be severe in all the domains for patients C and D. Table 1 summarizes the scores achieved by the children.

Cognitive level: Cognitive assessment at baseline resulted in low normal MDI for patient B, while patients C and D had significant cognitive delays. Cognitive assessment was not completed for patient A for lack of cooperation; still he reached average scores on the subtests that he did perform. After one year of intervention, patient A had normal and patient B above normal cognitive abilities. Patients C and D continued to have significant cognitive delays.

Language: Following one year of intervention, patients A and B had 3-4 word utterances, used verbs as well as other grammatical markers and were able to answer simple questions. Patients C and D had a limited vocabulary that did not exceed five clear words that were used inconsistently. In addition, they did not combine words and had poor understanding. By Schuler's definition (1976; cited in Fay, 1980), patients B and C were non-verbal.

Table 1. Scores on the ADI, ADOS, the Bailey Scales and the Stanford-Binet during the first (I), and the second (II) evaluation of patients A, B, C and D

Time	Test	Patient	A	B	C	D
I	*ADI	Reciprocal Social Interaction	26	15	26	25
		Communication	18	8	14	14
		Repetitive Behaviors and Stereotyped Patterns	4	5	7	3
I	ADOS	New algorithm	***19	**19	**25	**25
I	Bailey	MDI	---	88	50	60
II	ADOS	New algorithm	#12	#11	*** 20	**23
II	Stanford-Binet	IQ	95	115	61	68

*ADI: Social interaction – cutoff >10; Communication - cutoff >7; Stereotypic behavior - cutoff >3.

**ADOS-Module 1 no words: cutoff for autism >16; autism spectrum >11.

***ADOS-Module 1 some words: cutoff for autism >12; autism spectrum >8.

#ADOS-Module 2 younger, new algorithm: cutoff points for autism >10; for autism spectrum >7.

Imaging: All patients demonstrated normal gray/white matter differentiation, normal midline structures to include corpus callosum, cavum septum pellucidum, pituitary gland and chiasm, normal cerebellum, vermis and cranio-cervical junction. None of the patients demonstrated cortical dysgenesis.

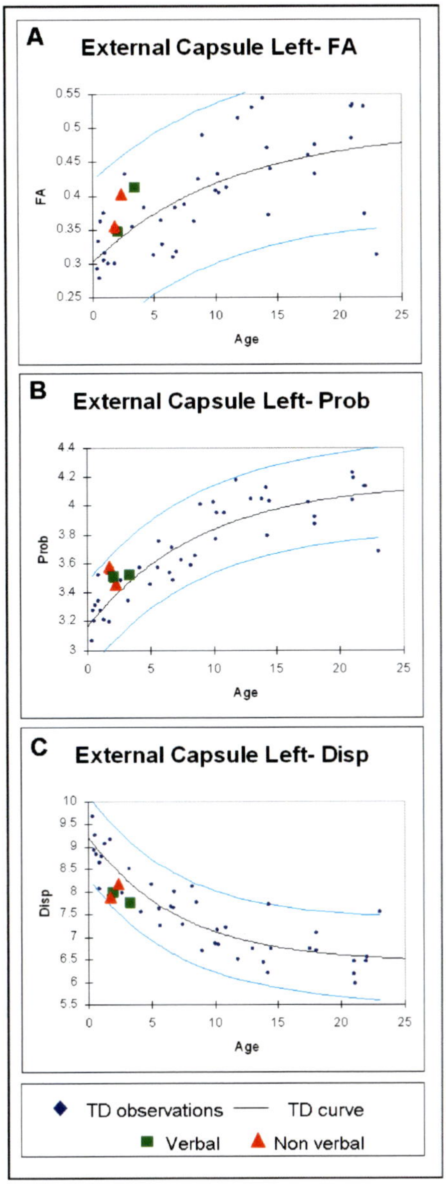

Figure 2. Data obtained from the left external capsule (left ec). Typical developmental curves were obtained using minimal regression analysis. Values of FA is presented in A, Prob is presented in B and Disp is presented in C. FA and prob values are measured in arbitrary units (a.u.), disp is measured in micrometers (μm). Individual values of all three indices are plotted against the predicted developmental curve for TD subjects.

In the overall WMPC analysis, all values were within the confidence interval, yet the Displacement values recorded for the four children were above the mean values of the control group. No differences in WMPC were detected between patients A and B who developed language, and patients C and D who remained non-verbal.

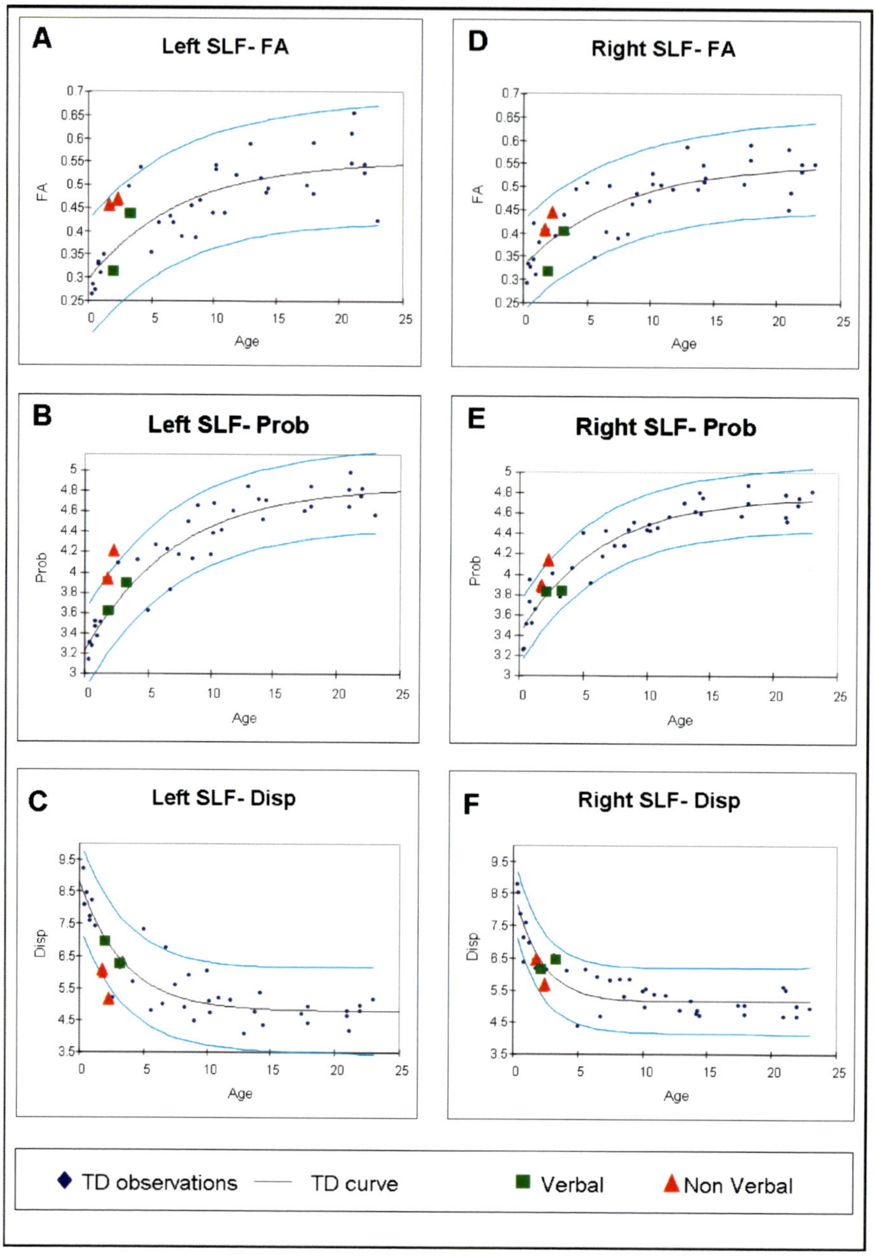

Figure 3. Data obtained from the left (A-C), and right (D-F) superior longitudinal fasciculus (slf) regions. Typical developmental curves were obtained using minimal regression analysis showing values of FA, Prob and Disp. FA and prob values are measured in arbitrary units (a.u.), and disp is measured in micrometers (μm). Individual values of all three indices are plotted against the predicted developmental curve for TD subjects.

All the participants were above the developmental curve on the diffusivity measures in the following brain areas: posterior, external capsule-left and forceps minor-left.

Prob was increased and Disp was decreased with no differences in the FA values in the anterior limb of the internal capsule -left and right, fminor-right and cortico-spinal-tracts-left in slice 3. However, values in these areas did not distinguish between patients A and B, and C and D. Figure 2 demonstrates the results seen for the external capsule.

Differences between patients A and B, and patients C and D who remained non-verbal and were cognitively impaired, were noted in the left-SLF in all three indices - Probability (prob), Displacement (Disp) and FA. Figure 3 demonstrates those results. Prob and Disp values of patients C and D, who remained non-verbal, were outside the 95% confidence interval for TD children of the same age.

FA values, although not strictly outside the confidence level, showed a similar trend. Such differences were not seen in the right-SLF, where measures of diffusivities did not differ between patients A and B (verbal), and patients C and D (non-verbal).

No significant differences between patients A and B and patients C and D and children in the control group were detected in the gray matter inferior frontal gyrus.

Discussion

While the clinical presentation of the children at the time of the MRI was not significantly different, prominent pre-intervention brain abnormalities were apparent between patients who, following one year of intervention remained non-verbal, and those who acquired language. Importantly, those were confined to the left -SLF which subserves the neuronal populations of the language areas.

These results are in line with previous studies of several developmental disorders which reported correlation between white matter integrity in the SLFand language and cognitive abilities (31).

For example, performance in visuospatial abilities in Williams syndrome (32); language performance in schizophrenia (33) and reading abilities in typically developing children (34,35) were all associated with white matter abnormalities.

Whereas it is tempting to relate the current results to the children's language status, such an interpretation is not without problems. Thus, although the significant cognitive deficits documented in the non-verbal boys were expected to correlate with structural abnormalities of the gray matter language areas, we did not find differences in restriction values in these areas. Lack of significant changes in the gray matter could originate from several technical limitations. Factors such as partial volume-effect, or the fact that the regions of interest were defined anatomically from the MRI rather than functionally selected from fMRI, might explain the negative results. Alternatively, it may reflect the fact that gray matter areas are less restricted compartments, and consequently DTI is not sensitive enough and does not detect subtle changes in these regions.

An additional problem concerns the fact that patients A and B differed from patients C and D not only in their language but in their autism severity at time II as well. It is therefore possible that differences in white matter integrity were related to the autism symptoms rather than to language per se. Alternatively, the status of language may be related to autism severity and to whatever biological cause was responsible for it. However, the fact that structural differences were confined to the left-SLF highlights the correlation of these results to the language status of the patients. We would therefore like to propose the hypothesis that white matter abnormality of the left-slf may predict the potential for language development in autism.

Importantly, these results leave open questions regarding the origin of the pathopysiology of autism. It is not clear whether this is a primary or a secondary process of neuronal alteration. If the abnormal structure of the left-slf, adjoining Broca's and Wernicke's areas, is conceived as evidence of precocious maturation, it might suggest that its adverse effect on the function of this fiber tract is due to the fact that connected areas have not followed a similar pace.

In conclusion, our findings highlight the involvement of issues of timing of developmental processes in the pathology of autism. It enhances the view of the brain as a network, whose normal functioning is dependent upon inherent structural integrity, along with coordinated developmental events (22).

Such a view suggests that abnormal local maturation can potentially create disequilibrium which could threaten to disrupt the operation of the network and prevent it from achieving normal functioning.

Acknowledgments

This work was supported by the March of Dimes grant 12-FY05-58. We gratefully acknowledge the co-operation of the children and their families.

Appendix

Case descriptions

Patient A

A was first diagnosed with autism at the age of 2;10 years, when he was referred for assessment of developmental regression, arrest of speech and accumulating autistic symptoms. A used gestures and pointing, had single words at the age of 1;.01, and two words combinations when he was 1.6. When A was two, he stopped using language for communication and his speech became echolalic. Cognitive assessment was only partially completed for lack of cooperation, but was assumed to be close to normal. Medical history was unremarkable. EEG, metabolic tests and an MRI obtained to assess his developmental regression were all normal.

A had a second evaluation at the age of four, following one year of intervention. A improved in his socio-communication skills but social interactions with other children remained problematic. He expressed his needs verbally, using appropriate questions and answers of three-four words long. A used tenses and inflectional morphology correctly and there was no echolalic speech. Cognitive level was found to be within the normal range (see Table 1).

Patient B

B was 1;11 years old when he was diagnosed with autism after being referred for assessment of poor eye contact and delayed communication. Family history was positive for anxiety, speech delay and autism. At the time of his diagnosis, receptive language was slightly delayed, and expressive language was severely impaired with no intelligible words. Assessment of cognitive ability revealed slightly below average level. Medical history was unremarkable but gross neurological examination revealed central hypotonia, for which he had an MRI performed at age 2;.0.

The second evaluation was obtained when B was 3;0, upon completion of the first year of intervention. B has improved significantly in his socio-communication skills. B produced three-four word utterances that included inflected verbs and other grammatical features and was able to maintain simple, short conversations. B incorporated immediate and delayed bits of echolalia into his free speech. Assessment of cognitive ability revealed above average performance (see Table 1).

Patient C

C was 2;0 years old when he was diagnosed with autism after referral for evaluation, because of severe developmental and communication delays. C had clear autistic symptoms as well as other behavioral problems (screaming, irritability, tantrums). C had sensory dysregulation (sensitivity to noise, sucking and mouthing objects). He was diagnosed with global developmental delay, most clearly manifested in the absence of language. Medical history revealed C had gastro-esophageal reflux resulting in frequent vomiting and his appetite was severely restricted.

Family history was positive for significant consanguinity of parents and grandparents and several individuals with severe mental retardation, autistic symptoms, seizures and aggressive behaviors. Neurological examination revealed moderate hypotonia, mild non-specific dysmorphism, few (less than 5) congenital hypo-and hyper pigmented skin spots. Hearing, vision, EEG, echocardiogram and basic metabolic and genetic tests were all normal. MRI was performed as part of a comprehensive evaluation of his significant delays.

A second evaluation was performed when C was 3;8 after completing a year of intensive intervention. At that time he could say five words and could follow very simple commands. Thus, language was still absent. C continued to have significant autism symptoms, including stereotypic behaviors and sensory dysregualtion. Assessment of cognitive ability revealed persistent significant delays (see Table 1).

Patient D

D was diagnosed with autism when he was 2.0 after being referred for evaluation of poor eye contact, repetitive behaviors, excessive sensory interests and poor communication. D had significant autistic symptoms, lack of pointing and very limited primary gestures. He produced very few sounds, and those were not directed to others. Excessive visual sensory stimulation, motor mannerism and stereotypic play (twirling objects and throwing toys) were noted. D had moderate to severe delays in fine motor development.

D did not understand simple verbal commands and could produce only infrequent syllables. Cognitive assessment revealed below average abilities. Neurological examination was intact except for head circumference > 97 percentile. Genetic and metabolic tests were negative. To further evaluate his macrocephaly and moderate to severe developmental delays, an MRI was performed.

D had a second evaluation when he was 3;.11 after completing one year of intervention. D continued to have severe socio-communication deficits and strong sensory interests, mannerism, flapping of his arms and turning around continuously. D produced many sounds several of which were word approximations, but no clear words. D had no conventional gestures, occasionally used pointing, but mostly used other people's hands to communicate his intentions. Cognitive evaluation revealed persistent significant delays (see Table 1).

References

[1] Ben Itzchak E, Lahat E, Burgin R, Zachor DA. Cognitive, behavior and intervention outcome correlates in young children with autism. Res. Dev. Disabi. 2008;29:447-58.

[2] Rapin I, Dunn M. Update on the language disorders of individuals on the autistic spectrum. Brain Dev. 2003;25:166-72.

[3] Wilcox J, Tsuang M, Ledger E, Algeo J, Schnurr T. Brain perfusion in autism varies with age. Neuropsychobiology 2002;46:13-6.

[4] Herbert MR, Ziegler DA, Deutsch CK, O'Brien LM, Kennedy DN, Filipek PA, et al. Brain asymmetries in autism and developmental language disorder: a nested whole-brain analysis. Brain 2005;128(Pt 1): 213-26.

[5] Flagg EJ, Cardy JE, Roberts W, Roberts TP. Language lateralization development in children with autism: insights form the late field magnetoencephalogram. Neurosci. Lett. 2005;386:82-7.

[6] De Fossé L, Hodge SM, Makris N, Kennedy D N, Caviness VS, McGrath L, et al. Language-association cortex asymmetry in autism and specific language impairment. Ann. Neurol. 2004;56:755-6.

[7] Redcay E, Courchesne E. Deviant functional magnetic resonance imaging patterns of brain activity to speech in 2-3-year-old children with autism spectrum disorder. Biol. Psychiatry 2008;64:589-98.

[8] Cascio CJ, Gerig G, Piven J. Diffusion tensor imaging: Application to the study of the developing brain. J. Am. Acad. Child Adolesc. Psychiatry 2007; 46:213-23.

[9] Mukherjee P, Miller JH, Shimony JS, Conturo TE, Lee BC, Almli CR, et al. Normal brain maturation during childhood: developmental trends characterized with diffusion-tensor MR imaging. Radiology 2001;221:349-58.

[10] Schmithorst VJ, Wilke M, Dardzinski BJ, Holland SK. (): Correlation of white matter diffusivity and anisotropy with age during childhood and adolescence: a cross-sectional diffusion-tensor MR imaging study. Radiology 2002;222:212-8.

[11] Dubois J, Dehaene-Lambertz G, Perrin M, Mangin JF, Cointepas Y, Duchesnay E, Le Bihan D, Hertz-Pannier L. Asynchrony of the early maturation of white matter bundles in healthy infants: quantitative landmarks revealed noninvasively by diffusion tensor imaging. Hum. Brain Mapp. 2008;29:14-27.

[12] Mukherjee P, McKinstry RC. Diffusion tensor imaging and tractography of human brain development. Neuroimaging Clin. N. Am. 2006;16:19-43.

[13] Assaf Y, Cohen Y. Assignment of the water slow-diffusing component in the central nervous system using q-space diffusion MRS: implications for fiber tract imaging. Magn. Reson. Med. 2000; 43:191-9.

[14] Ben-Bashat D, Ben Sira L, Graif, M, Pianka P, Hendler T, Cohen Y, et al. White matter maturation from birth through adulthood: high b value diffusion weighted imaging study. In: Ng V, Barker GJ, Hendler T, eds. Structural MRI in Psychiatry, Psychiatric Neuroimaging, Amsterdam: IOS Press, 2003.

[15] Ben Bashat D, Ben Sira L, Graif M, Pianka P, Hendler T, Cohen Y, et al. Normal white matter development from infancy to adulthood: comparing diffusion tensor and high b value diffusion weighted MR images. J. Magn. Reson. Imaging 2005:21:503-511.

[16] DeLano MC, Cao Y. High b-value diffusion imaging. Neuroimaging Clin. N. Am. 2002;12:21-34.

[17] Barnea-Goraly N, Kwon H, Menon V, Eliez S, Lotspeich L, Reiss AL. White matter structure in autism: preliminary evidence from diffusion tensor imaging. Biol. Psychiatry 2004;55:323-6.

[18] Alexander A, Lee J, Lazar M, Boudos R, Dubray M, Oakes T, et al. Diffusion tensor imaging of the corpus callosum in Autism. Neuroimage 2007;34:61-73.

[19] Sundaram SK, Kumar A, Makki MI, Behen ME, Chugani HT, Chugani DC. Diffusion Tensor Imaging of Frontal Lobe in Autism Spectrum Disorder. Cereb. Cortex 2008;11:2659-65.

[20] Ben Bashat D, Kronfeld-Duenias V, Zachor D, Ekstein P, Hendler T, Tarrasch R, et al. Accelerated maturation of white matter in young children. Neuroimage 2007;37:40-7.

[21] Weinstein, M., Ben-Sira, L., Levy, Y., Zachor, D. A., Ben Itzhak, E., Arzi, M., Tarrasch, R., Ekstein, P. M, Hendler, T. & Ben Bashat, D. (2011) Abnormal white matter structure in young children with autism. Human Brain Mapping, 32(4), 534-543

[22] Courchesne E, Pierce K. Brain overgrowth in autism during a critical time in development: implications for frontal pyramidal neuron and interneuron development and connectivity. Int. J. Dev. Neurosci, 2005; 23:153-70.

[23] Muller R. The study of autism as a distributed disorder. Ment. Retard Dev. Disabil Res. Rev., 2007;13:85-95.

[24] Lord C, Rutter M, Le Couteur A. Autism Diagnostic Interview-Revised: a revised version of a diagnostic interview for caregivers of individuals with possible pervasive developmental disorders. J. Autism Dev. Disord. 1994;24:659-85.

[25] Lord C, Rutter M, DiLavore PC, Risi S. Autism Diagnostic Observation Schedule-WPS (ADOS-WPS). Los Angeles: Western Psychol. Serv., 1999.

[26] American Psychiatric Association. Diagnostic and statistical manual of mental disorders (DSM-IV), 4th ed. Washington, DC: Author, 1994.

[27] Bayley N. Bayley Scales for Infant Development – second edition manual. San Antonio, TX: Psychol. Corp., 1993.

[28] Gotham K, Risi, S, Dawson G, Tager-Flusberg H, Joseph R, Carter A, et al. A replication of the Autism Diagnostic Observation Schedule (ADOS) revised algorithms. J. Am. Acad. child Adolesc. Psychiatry 2008;47:642-651.

[29] Thorndike RL, Hagen E. Sattler J. Stanford-Binet Intelligence Scale, 4th, ed. Itasca, Ill: Riverside, 1986.

[30] Fay WH. Aspects of speech. In: Fay AL, Emerging language in autistic children. Baltimore, MD: Univ. Park Press, 1980.

[31] Mori S, Wakana S, Nagae-Postscher L, M, van Zijl PCM. MRI Atlas of Human White Matter. Amsterdam: Elsevier BV, 2005.

[32] Dubois J, Hertz-Pannier L, Cachia A, Mangin JF, Le Bihan D, Dehaene-Lambertz G. Structural asymmetries in the infant language and sensori-motor networks. Cereb. Cortex 2009;19:414-23.

[33] Hoeft F, Barnea-Goraly N, Haas BW, Golarai G, Ng D, Mills D, Korenberg J, Bellugi U, Galaburda A, Reiss AL. More is not always better: increased fractional anisotropy of superior longitudinal fasciculus associated with poor visuospatial abilities in Williams syndrome. J. Neurosci. 2007;31(27):11960-5.

[34] Karlsgodt KH, Sun D, Jimenez AM, Lutkenhoff ES, Willhite R, Van Erp TG, Cannon TD. Developmental disruptions in neural connectivity in the pathophysiology of schizophrenia. Dev. Psychopathol. 2008;20:1297-327.

[35] Beaulieu C, Plewes C, Paulson LA, Roy D, Snook L, Concha L, Phillips L. Imaging brain connectivity in children with diverse reading ability. Neuroimage 2005;25:1266-71.

[36] Deutsch GK, Dougherty RF, Bammer R, Siok WT, Gabrieli JD, Wandell B. Children's reading performance is correlated with white matter structure measured by diffusion tensor imaging. Cortex 2005; 41:354-63.

In: Understanding Autism Spectrum Disorder
Editors: Ditza A Zachor and Joav Merrick

ISBN: 978-1-62081-353-9

Chapter 13

Intact cognitive flexibility in parents of autistic children

Esther Vierck*, Abraham Reichenberg, Philip D. Harvey and Jeremy M. Silverman
Department of Psychiatry, Mount Sinai School of Medicine, New York, US,
Department of Psychological Medicine, Institute of Psychiatry, King's College, London and Emory University School of Medicine, Atlanta, Georgia, US

Abstract

Autism is a genetically complex disorder. Determining individualized phenotypic elements (i.e. endophenotypes) of the broader autism phenotype in first-degree family members of autistic children may facilitate the search for associated genes through molecular genetic studies. Executive functions have been suggested as such endophenotypes. Set-shifting/switching in first-degree relatives has mainly been investigated with the Wisconsin Card Sorting Test, whereas switching within a verbal task has not been examined at all. Our objective was to examine set-shifting in a verbal and a non-verbal task setting in addition to planning abilities in parents of autistic children and a healthy control group. We conducted a cross-sectional case control study with 32 mothers and fathers of autistic children and an age matched control group consisting of 32 healthy adults. We used measures from the Delis-Kaplan Executive Function Scale. In particular, the Trail Making Test, a Verbal Fluency Task, and a Tower test were employed for assessment. Results: We found no evidence of a set-shifting/switching deficit in parents of autistic children. In addition, we observed no group differences in tests assessing verbal fluency planning performance. The results provide no support for set-shifting/cognitive flexibility as an endophenotype of autism.

* Correspondence: Esther Vierck, Department of Psychiatry, Mount Sinai School of Medicine, One Gustave L. Levy Place, New York, NY 10029, United States. Tel: +001 (212) 659-5656; Fax: +001 (212) 659-5626 ; E-mail: esther.vierck@mssm.edu

Introduction

Autism is a chronic developmental disorder characterized by deficits in social behavior, impairments in communication skills and language development, and repetitive, stereotyped behavior (1). Twin and family studies suggest that genetic factors are prominent in the etiology of the disorder (2). Family studies have also been conducted to explore the autism broader phenotype (3), that is, the existence of milder, subclinical, or varied expressions of characteristics associated with autism in non-autistic family members. The ultimate goal of these studies is to provide a clear definition of variables associated with autism, which would benefit genetic studies. Executive function deficits have been investigated as potential elements or endophenotypes of the broader autistic phenotype in previous research studies (4,5). Executive functions are associated with goal directed behavior, and include abilities such as planning, task switching, and mental flexibility. There is considerable evidence for executive deficits in autism (4,6), specifically impairments in planning (5,7), set-shifting (4,5,7) and verbal fluency (4,5) have been reported frequently, and have been proposed as core deficits in cognitive models of the disorder (8).

Research in family members is limited and inconsistent. Some studies reported planning deficits in parents of autistic children (3,9), while others found no evidence of such a deficit (10,11). Other abilities that may be impaired in first-degree relatives are set-shifting, working memory (9) and fluency (11), but these findings are not consistent (12). Overall, there are indications of at least some executive function deficits in some autism parents. Measures of mental flexibility and verbal fluency tasks have been shown to be impaired in autistic probands (4,6,13), but only a few studies have focused on whether these traits are also more evident in non-autistic relatives of autism probands.

In the present case-control study, we focused mainly on mental flexibility tasks and investigated whether the executive function deficits observed in autism probands in this area are also present in their parents. The overall goal is the isolation of endophenotypes associated with autism to facilitate future molecular genetic studies. Toward this end, we measured mental flexibility with non-verbal and verbal tasks, verbal fluency, and planning abilities in parents with autistic children. These measures were then compared to the performance of a healthy adult control group.

Our study

Thirty-two parents of autistic children (eight males) and 32 age but not gender matched control participants (13 males) selected out of the control subject pool of the Family Studies Research Center in New York City took part in this study. Autism families were recruited from the participant pool of the Family Studies Research Center in which trained research personal confirmed the diagnosis of the autistic child with the Autism Diagnostic Interview-Revised (14) and the Autism Diagnostic Observation Schedule-Generic (15).

Written consent was obtained following the guidelines of the Mount Sinai School of Medicine Human Subjects Research Committee. All the results reported below and the description of the demographic data of the autism parents and the controls summarized in table 1 are based on this random sample of 32 control participants.

Table 1. Descriptive data for autism parents and the control group

	Autism Parents	Controls	F/Chi^2	P value
Age (standard deviation) Males / Females	46.8 (9.17) 50.0 / 45.8	44.8 (9.85) 42.7 / 46.2	.328	.569
Gender (% male)	25%	40.63%	.287	.143
Ethnicity (% white)	65.63%	56% *	.761	.683
IQ (standard deviation) Males / Females	110.9 (15.40) 117.4 / 108.7	103.1 (16.07) 101.9 / 103.8	.369	.546

* 7 control participants did not declare their ethnicity.

Study population

Autism parents were on average slightly older than control parents, but this difference was not significant. A separate analysis for both genders revealed men in the control group to be on average 7.31 years younger than men in the autism group. This difference reached statistical significance ($t = -2.326$, $p = .031$). Control women were similar in age to the females in the autism group. The ethnic distribution between groups was also similar. Intelligence overall was slightly above average. The autism group seemed to have somewhat higher intelligence scores overall, but this difference was not statistically significant. Scores for IQ were similar when only women were compared. But there was a trend for fathers of autistic children to have higher IQ scores than control men ($p = .064$).

Neuropsychological assessments

Intelligence was assessed using the Wechsler Abbreviated Scale of Intelligence (WASI 16). In most cases the four-subtest version was used, but due to time limitations (14) of the autism parents were tested with the two-subtest version. Both versions provide very good estimates of general intelligence (16). We used the full-IQ measures resulting from either version of the WASI to create one overall intelligence variable for all participants.

Executive functions were assessed using the Delis-Kaplan Executive Function Scale (D-KEFS) (17). The D-KEFS provides not only measures of general performance but also several measures of process components, which are thought to underlie executive functions. We a-priori selected tests that assess switching abilities and planning. The Trail Making Test (TMT) and the verbal fluency Test, for the former, and the Tower Test for the latter.

TMT

The TMT is modified after the TMT in the Halstead-Reitan Neuropsychological Battery (18). Participants are required to connect circles on a sheet of paper in accordance to certain rules. It consists of five conditions with which visual scanning, visual-motor sequencing for numbers and letters, number-letter switching, and motor speed are measured. Among these the number-letter switching task is thought to be a measure of cognitive flexibility able to capture even subtle executive-function deficits (19). In this task participants are required to alternate between connecting sequences of letters and numbers. For all these tasks the time until task completion is recorded.

TMT process components

For the TMT we will also use a normed combined sequencing measure included in the D-KEFS manual, which is calculated from the letter and number sequencing scores. Combined scores increase the probability of detecting differences, especially in cases of across-test individual variability, which has been found previously (20). The measure used here allows us to investigate whether a general sequencing deficit independent of the stimuli used, might be present in parents of autistic probands.

Contrast measures are also normed variables of the D-KEFS scale. They allow a direct quantification of either a baseline measure and a higher function measure or between two higher function measures, for example, the contrast measure Number-Letter Switching vs.

Motor Speed measures switching abilities between numbers and letters adjusted by the influence of motor speed. These measures are calculated by subtraction of one scaled score from the other. This difference score is then converted to a new score, which has again a mean score of 10 and a standard deviation of 3. Because of this procedure under- and overestimations of executive function measures due to other factors are avoided (19).

Verbal fluency test

In the Verbal Fluency Task participants are asked to produce as many words as possible with each of the initial letters F, A, and S. In other conditions verbal categories are highlighted as names of animal species and boy's names have to be generated. In the final condition, participants have to alternate in the generation of fruits and pieces of furniture. In this last task verbal fluency and switching abilities are combined, which places a stronger demand on executive functions than the first two conditions. Each of the six conditions has a time frame of one minute for execution; measured are the number of responses generated and additionally the accuracy of responses for the switching task.

Tower test

The Tower test assesses planning abilities (19). This test is modified after the Tower of Hanoi (21). Participants are required to construct displayed target towers by moving disks of different sizes across three pegs, while following rules which specify what kind of moves are allowed. Nine target towers are provided; total achievement scores, which provide a global measure of performance, are reported here. Several executive functions are necessary for a good task performance.

Data analysis

We performed univariate Analysis of Covariance (ANCOVA) analysis with the factors group (autism parents vs. control parents) and gender (males vs. females). We used the Benjamini-Hochberg method (22) to prevent an increased risk of Type I errors due to multiple testing. All models included IQ as a covariate. Age was not used as a covariate because all variable scores used were already adjusted to age. The different variables investigated were the five measures of the TMT and the six compound and contrast measure variables, the four measures of the Verbal Fluency Test and their contrast measures, and the achievement score of the Tower Test. Based on our literature review we hypothesized performance deficits in the TMT switching condition, fluency and tower tasks for the autism parents relative to the performance of the control participants.

Pattern of missing data

Of 704 data points, nine (six from autism parents, three from controls) were missing (1.28%). Most of the missing data affected the IQ measurement (6). Due to an administration error only verbal and not performance IQ was measured in most of these cases. For two other participants scores of the Tower test were missing and for another participant, accuracy of the switching category in the verbal fluency task was accidentally not scored. It thus seems that the missing data was random. We substituted missing data through regression analysis with the group data to the values missing for all available data. To make sure that missing data had no influence, we conducted the analysis once with the missing data substituted as explained above and once with a reduced subject number, which resulted from the elimination of all missing data cases. This analysis did lead to slightly weaker results most likely due to the reduced number of participants. The data reported here is the data with the substituted values. We believe that the good fit achieved through regression analysis allows for a more realistic picture than the deletion of cases.

Our findings

The ANCOVA performed with the five variables of the TMT led to one significant result before the Benjamini-Hochberg correction; control participants performed better in the Number-Letter Switching condition of the TMT than autism parents this effect was not modified by gender, but after applying the Benjamini-Hochberg correction this difference became non-significant. The mean performance scores adjusted for IQ are displayed in table 2.

TMT process components

The ANCOVA performed with the six variables of the TMT process components lead to similar results. Before the Benjamini-Hochberg correction switching deficits in the performance of autism parents for the contrast measure of Number-Letter Switching vs. Motor Speed could be observed, but these effects vanished after the correction. Mean performance scores adjusted IQ for the TMT process components are displayed in table 3.

In addition, there was an effect of gender on the TMT process components.

The factors gender and group interacted for the contrast variable Number-Letter Switching vs. Visual Scanning ($F(1,59) = 4.58$, $p < 0.05$). But as before, the effect disappeared after the Benjamini-Hochberg correction. Overall, the findings of the TMT do not confirm our hypothesis. Our data provide no evidence for a switching deficit in autism parents.

Table 2. Performance (means and standard error in brackets) for the Trail Making Test as a function of group (autism parents vs. controls) and gender (male vs. female) after adjustment of IQ

	Autism Parents	Controls	F value	P value
Visual Scanning	10.97 (0.64)	11.59 (0.51)	.489	.487
Number Sequencing	9.81 (0.69)	10.29 (0.55)	.038	.845
Letter Sequencing	9.59 (0.61)	10.16 (0.49)	.569	.453
Number-Letter Switching	10.00 (0.50)	11.29 (0.40)	5.544	.022
Motor Speed	10.19 (0.75)	9.40 (0.60)	1.213	.275

Table 3. Performance (means and standard error in brackets) for the Trail Making Test process components as a function of group (autism parents vs. controls) and gender (male vs. female) after adjustment of IQ

	Autism Parents	Controls	F/Chi^2	P value
Combined Number Sequencing + Letter Sequencing	10.42 (0.54)	10.64 (0.47)	.090	.765
Number-Letter Switching vs. Visual Scanning	9.19 (0.45)	9.91 (0.39)	1.381	.245
Number-Letter Switching vs. Number Sequencing	10.05 (0.54)	11.05 (0.47)	1.885	.175
Number-Letter Switching vs. Letter Sequencing	10.34 (0.53)	11.14 (0.46)	1.253	.268
Number-Letter Switching vs. Combined Number sequencing + Letter sequencing	9.63 (0.52)	10.68 (0.45)	2.229	.141
Number-Letter Switching vs. Motor Speed	9.82 (0.60)	12.04 (0.52)	7.466	.008

Verbal fluency

Our analysis revealed no effects of group or gender on any variable of the Verbal Fluency conditions. The performance data adjusted for IQ for the variables of this test are displayed in table 4.

Table 4. Performance (means and standard error in brackets) for the Verbal Fluency Test and the Tower Test as a function of group (autism parents vs. controls) and gender (male vs. female) after adjustment of IQ

	Autism Parents	Controls	F/Chi^2	P value
Letter Fluency	11.39 (0.80)	11.06 (0.70)	.90	.765
Category Fluency	11.61 (0.65)	10.87 (0.57)	.703	.405
Category Switching Total Correct Responses	10.67 (0.75)	11.41 (0.65)	.528	.470
Category Switching Total Switching Accuracy	10.88 (0.73)	11.40 (0.64)	.281	.598
Tower Test	9.57 (0.51)	9.93 (0.44)	.281	.598

Planning

We were unable to replicate any planning impairment. There were no performance differences between groups for the Tower test. In a further analysis, we separated the individual tower trials to easy (1-3 moves) and difficult (more that 3 moves) because a previous investigation reported impairments only in more difficult task situations 7.

Again, we found no significant differences in our analysis. This indicates that at least for our sample planning deficits are not present in the parents of autism probands. The performance data adjusted for IQ for this test is also displayed in table 4.

Discussion

In a cross-sectional case control study, we failed to demonstrate executive function deficits in parents of autistic children. In particular, we investigated set shifting/cognitive flexibility abilities, verbal fluency and planning skills and found for none of these measures performance differences between first-degree relatives of autistic children and a healthy control group. These results are in line with other studies that also found no deficits for the assessed functions (10-12). Our results thus suggest that the cognitive function of set-shifting may not be part of the broader autism phenotype.

Some studies reported set-shifting/cognitive flexibility difficulties in relatives of autistic probands (9, 23). In these cases a version of the Wisconsin Card Sorting Test (WCST) (24) has been used. In contrast, one study, that like us used the switching subset of the TMT, reported also no set-shifting deficit (25). This pattern of results suggests that different findings may be due to differences in task difficulty. In the WCST tasks shifts are much harder to detect than in our verbal and non-verbal assessment, where shifts occur predictably after each item. This possibility is supported by findings that indicate an influence of task difficulty on performance in autistic children (7). It is conceivable that task difficulty also affects first-degree relatives of autistic children.

The current study has several limitations. First, the autistic probands were not assessed on the neuropsychological tests. Data like this would allow tracking of deficits within families. Unfortunately, the neuropsychological tests used were too demanding for most of autistic children. Second, healthy siblings of the autistic proband were also not assessed. It is possible that some executive function deficits are more pronounced in children as executive functions develop. Third, the small number of fathers made the analysis of a gender effect difficult. Fourth, our failure to find differences between parents of children with autism and healthy controls is associated with our correction for multiple comparisons. This correction conservatively decreased the p-value used in the assessment of significance. Together with the diversity commonly found in autism spectrum disorder, this might have influenced our results. Lastly, in contrast to most other studies within this area our control group consisted of healthy controls. In the majority of studies autism relatives have been compared to relatives of children with other disorders than autism. The advantage of such a control group is that parents share the same "burden of care", which might impact on test performance. It is also useful in finding specific autistic traits. On the other hand some of the traits under investigation may not only be impaired in autism, but also in other disorders that otherwise have no connection to autism. Such a scenario would make it more difficult to isolate autistic endophenotypes.

Conclusion

Our study contributes to the growing knowledge regarding the broader autism phenotype by suggesting that the function of set-shifting/cognitive flexibility is intact in parents of autistic children and thus not part of the endophenotype of autism.

Acknowledgments

This study was supported by a Young Investigator Award from Cure Autism Now (currently Autism Speaks) to A. Reichenberg, grant support from the Beatrice and Samuel A. Seaver Foundation to Vierck and Silverman, and the National Institutes of Health (MH-066673). During the past year, Dr. Harvey has served as a consultant to: Eli Lilly and Company, Johnson and Johnson, Dainippon Sumitomo America, Merck and Company, Pfizer, Wyeth Pharma, He has received grant support from: Astra-Zeneca. Dr. Vierck, Dr. Silverman, and Dr. Reichenberg reported no financial interest or potential conflicts of interest.

References

American Psychiatric Association. Diagnotic and Statistical Manual of Mental Disorder, Fourth Edition. Washington, DC: *APA*, 1994.

Barnard L, Muldoon K, Hasan R, O'Brien G, Stewart M. Profiling executive dysfunction in adults with autism and comorbid learning disability. *Autism* 2008;12(2):125-41.

Benjamini Y, Hochberg T. Controlling the False Discovery Rate: a practical and powerful approach to multiple testing. *J. Royal Stat. Soc. B.* 1995;85:289–300.

Borys SV, Spitz HH, Dorans BA. Tower of Hanoi performance of retarded young adults and nonretarded children as a function of solution length and goal state. *J. Exp. Child Psychol.* 1982;33(1):87-110.

Delis DC, and Kaplan, E. Delis-Kaplan Executive Function Scale. San Antonio, TX: *Psychol. Corp.*, 2001.

Delis DC, Kaplan, E., and Kramer, J. H. Delis–Kaplan executive function system technical manual. San Antonio, TX*: Psychol. Corp.*, 2001.

Delorme R, Gousse V, Roy I, Trandafir A, Mathieu F, Mouren-Simeoni MC, Betancur C, Leboyer M. Shared executive dysfunctions in unaffected relatives of patients with autism and obsessive-compulsive disorder. *Eur. Psychiatry* 2007;22(1):32-8.

Delorme R, Goussé V, Roy I, Trandafir A, Mathieu F, Mouren-Siméoni MC, Betancur C, Leboyer M. Shared executive dysfunctions in unaffected relatives of patients with autism and obsessive-compulsive disorder. *Eur. Psychiatry* 2007;22(1):32-8.

Grant DA, Berg EA. A behavioral analysis of degree of reinforcement and ease of shifting to new responses in a Weigl-type card-sorting problem. *J. Exp. Psychol.* 1948;38(4):404-11.

Hughes C, Leboyer M, Bouvard M. Executive function in parents of children with autism. *Psychol. Med.* 1997;27(1):209-20.

Hughes C, Plumet MH, Leboyer M. Towards a cognitive phenotype for autism: increased prevalence of executive dysfunction and superior spatial span amongst siblings of children with autism. *J. Child Psychol. Psychiatr.* 1999;40(5):705-18.

Hughes C, Russell J, Robbins TW. Evidence for executive dysfunction in autims. *Neuropsychologia* 1994;32(4):477-92.

Kleinhans N, Akshoomoff N, Delis DC. Executive functions in autism and Asperger's disorder: flexibility, fluency, and inhibition. *Dev. Neuropsychol.* 2005;27(3):379-401.

Lord C, Risi S, Lambrecht L, Cook EH, Jr., Leventhal BL, DiLavore PC, Pickles A, Rutter M. The autism diagnostic observation schedule-generic: a standard measure of social and communication deficits associated with the spectrum of autism. *J. Autism Dev. Disord.* 2000;30(3):205-23.

Lord C, Rutter M, Le Couteur A. Autism Diagnostic Interview-Revised: a revised version of a diagnostic interview for caregivers of individuals with possible pervasive developmental disorders. *J. Autism Dev. Disord.* 1994;24(5):659-85.

Minshew NJ, Williams DL. The new neurobiology of autism: cortex, connectivity, and neuronal organization. *Arch. Neurol.* 2007;64(7):945-50.

Prior M, Hoffmann W. Brief report: neuropsychological testing of autistic children through an exploration with frontal lobe tests. *J. Autism Dev. Disord.* 1990;20(4):581-90.

Psychological Corporation. Wechsler abbreviated scale of intelligence manual. San Antonio, TX: *Harcourt Brace*,1999.

Reitan RM, Wolfson, D. Halstead-Reitan Neuropsychological Battery. Tuscon, AZ: *Neuropsychol Press*, 1993.

Rumsey JM, Hamburger SD. Neuropsychological findings in high-functioning men with infantile autism, residual state. *J. Clin. Exp. Neuropsychol.* 1988;10(2):201-21.

Silverman JM, Smith CJ, Schmeidler J, Hollander E, Lawlor BA, Fitzgerald M, Buxbaum JD, Delaney K, Galvin P. Symptom domains in autism and related conditions: evidence for familiality. *Am. J. Med. Genet.* 2002;114(1):64-73.

Szatmari P, Jones MB, Tuff L, Bartolucci G, Fisman S, Mahoney W. Lack of cognitive impairment in first-degree relatives of children with pervasive developmental disorders. *J. Am. Acad. Child Adolesc. Psychiatry* 1993;32(6):1264-73.

Turner RA, Altemus M, Enos T, Cooper B, McGuinness T. Preliminary research on plasma oxytocin in normal cycling women: investigating emotion and interpersonal distress. *Psychiatry* 1999;62(2):97-113.

Verte S, Geurts HM, Roeyers H, Oosterlaan J, Sergeant JA. Executive functioning in children with autism and Tourette syndrome. *Dev. Psychopathol.* 2005;17(2):415-45.

Wong D, Maybery M, Bishop DV, Maley A, Hallmayer J. Profiles of executive function in parents and siblings of individuals with autism spectrum disorders. *Genes. Brain Behav.* 2006;5(8):561-76.

Section two: Acknowledgments

Chapter 14

About the editors

Ditza A Zachor, MD, graduated from the Technion Medical School in Israel, specialized and board certified in pediatrics, pediatric neurology and neuro-developmental disabilities at the Brown University in Providence, Rhode Island, United States. Served as the Director of Medical Services and assistant professor at the University of Alabama at Birmingham, Alabama, United States. Currently, senior lecturer at the Sackler School of Medicine, Tel Aviv University and the director of the Autism Center at the Assaf HaRofeh Medical Center, in Zerifin, Israel. Basic science research focused on the effects of drugs on neuronal signaling and clinical research on developmental medicine. Many recent papers published in the autism field mainly on intervention approaches, predictors of outcome, brain imaging and epidemiology of autism. E-mail: dzachor@asaf.health.gov.il

Joav Merrick, MD, MMedSci, DMSc, is professor of pediatrics, child health and human development affiliated with Kentucky Children's Hospital, University of Kentucky, Lexington, United States and the Division of Pediatrics, Hadassah Hebrew University Medical Centers, Mt Scopus Campus, Jerusalem, Israel, the medical director of the Health Services, Division for Intellectual and Developmental Disabilities, Ministry of Social Affairs and Social Services, Jerusalem, the founder and director of the National Institute of Child Health and Human Development in Israel. Numerous publications in the field of pediatrics, child health and human development, rehabilitation, intellectual disability, disability, health, welfare, abuse, advocacy, quality of life and prevention. Received the Peter Sabroe Child Award for outstanding work on behalf of Danish Children in 1985 and the International LEGO-Prize ("The Children's Nobel Prize") for an extraordinary contribution towards improvement in child welfare and well-being in 1987. E-mail: jmerrick@zahav.net.il

Chapter 15

About the Center for Autism, Assaf HaRofeh Medical Center, Zerifin, Israel

Assaf Harofeh Medical Center with the close collaboration of ALUT, The Israeli National Association for Children with Autism decided in 2002 to establish the Autism Center to promote autism care and research in Israel. The Autism Center serves as a national resource center for diagnosis, treatment and research in Autism Spectrum Disorders (ASD). The center has a goal to serve as an address for all aspects of ASD over the lifespan. This broad focus enables an easy flow of information and enrichment between professionals and researchers.

The Autism Center offers a unique opportunity to address the complex needs of children with ASD/autism. The center provides very early diagnosis for children from all over the State of Israel using the most advanced diagnostic instruments available. The diagnosis process includes comprehensive neurological assessment and use of state-of the-art autism diagnostic tools. Parents receive detailed description of the child's evaluation results and recommendations for medical diagnostic tests and treatment options.

Other services include follow-up assessments of the child's progress with intervention, Behavior consultations for complex and different behavior problems commonly occurring in autism/ASD, including assessment, analysis and guidance.

The center provides medical consultation for possible use of medication for children with complex behavioral and medical problems through the pharmacology clinic.

Early intervention

The center is also involved in early intervention in ASD. The early identification of children opens a window of opportunity to affect brain development, based on the critical time period of brain plasticity, by intervention and thereby building new neuronal pathways. Currently, the Autism Center provides medical supervision for many community autism-specific nurseries, and autism-specific kindergartens around the country. The early intervention preschool program at the Autism Center located at Assaf Harofeh hospital serves as a model program for experimental educational treatment. Then, based on the outcome and experience gathered in this model, the new strategies are implemented in other intervention programs that ALUT operates. The effectiveness of these programs has been examined by research and several papers were published on this topic in major peer-review journals.

The Autism Center provides comprehensive treatment services for adults. An individualized plan based on applied behavioral analysis principles focuses on improving the person's adaptive skills, communication and language and on decreasing behavior problems. A multi-disciplinary team including a senior behavior analyst, psychologist, social worker, speech and language pathologist and occupational therapist work in concert to achieve these goals.

The center is involved in creating and supervising courses related to autism in universities and colleges and training professionals in diagnosing ASD. In addition, the Autism Center serves as a tertiary center for consultation on children with complex clinical and behavioral presentation.

Research

As advances in neuroscience, molecular biology, genetics, pharmacology and behavioral sciences are making inroads into understanding autism; the center draws from all these disciplines to conduct collaborative research with various academic institutions in Israel and abroad. The center is involved in various research projects. The diagnostic facility evaluates a wide variety of children on the autism spectrum with different severity of symptoms, cognitive abilities, adaptive skills and medical problems. Many basic science and clinical research that might improve the diagnostic process and the intervention strategies are in progress. Currently, research has been both with in-house researchers as primary investigators and in collaboration with other hospitals and universities.

Contact

Ditza A Zachor, MD, Director
The Autism Center
Assaf HaRofeh Medical Center
Sackler School of Medicine
IL-70300 Zerifin, Israel
E-mail: dzachor@asaf.health.gov.il

Chapter 16

About the National Institute of Child Health and Human Development in Israel

The National Institute of Child Health and Human Development (NICHD) in Israel was established in 1998 as a virtual institute under the auspicies of the Medical Director, Ministry of Social Affairs and Social Services in order to function as the research arm for the Office of the Medical Director. In 1998 the National Council for Child Health and Pediatrics, Ministry of Health and in 1999 the Director General and Deputy Director General of the Ministry of Health endorsed the establishment of the NICHD. In 2011 the NICHD became affiliated with the Division of Pediatrics, Hadassah Hebrew University Medical Centers, Mt Scopus Campus in Jerusalem.

Mission

The mission of a National Institute for Child Health and Human Development in Israel is to provide an academic focal point for the scholarly interdisciplinary study of child life, health, public health, welfare, disability, rehabilitation, intellectual disability and related aspects of human development. This mission includes research, teaching, clinical work, information and public service activities in the field of child health and human development.

Service and academic activities

Over the years many activities became focused in the south of Israel due to collaboration with various professionals at the Faculty of Health Sciences (FOHS) at the Ben Gurion University of the Negev (BGU). Since 2000 an affiliation with the Zusman Child Development Center at the Pediatric Division of Soroka University Medical Center has resulted in collaboration around the establishment of the Down Syndrome Clinic at that center. In 2002 a full course on "Disability" was established at the Recanati School for Allied Professions in the Community, FOHS, BGU and in 2005 collaboration was started with the Primary Care Unit of the faculty and disability became part of the master of public health course on "Children and society". In the academic year 2005-2006 a one semester course on "Aging with disability" was started as part of the master of science program in gerontology in our collaboration with the Center for Multidisciplinary Research in Aging. In 2010 collaborations with the Division of Pediatrics, Hadassah Medical Centers, Hebrew University, Jerusalem, Israel.

Research activities

The affiliated staff have over the years published work from projects and research activities in this national and international collaboration. In the year 2000 the International Journal of Adolescent Medicine and Health and in 2005 the International Journal on Disability and Human development of De Gruyter Publishing House (Berlin and New York), in the year 2003 the TSW-Child Health and Human Development and in 2006 the TSW-Holistic Health and Medicine of the Scientific World Journal (New York and Kirkkonummi, Finland), all peer-reviewed international journals were affiliated with the National Institute of Child Health and Human Development. From 2008 also the International Journal of Child Health and Human Development (Nova Science, New York), the International Journal of Child and Adolescent Health (Nova Science) and the Journal of Pain Management (Nova Science) affiliated and from 2009 the International Public Health Journal (Nova Science) and Journal of Alternative Medicine Research (Nova Science).

National collaborations

Nationally the NICHD works in collaboration with the Faculty of Health Sciences, Ben Gurion University of the Negev; Department of Physical Therapy, Sackler School of Medicine, Tel Aviv University; Autism Center, Assaf HaRofeh Medical Center; National Rett and PKU Centers at Chaim Sheba Medical Center, Tel HaShomer; Department of Physiotherapy, Haifa University; Department of Education, Bar Ilan University, Ramat Gan, Faculty of Social Sciences and Health Sciences; College of Judea and Samaria in Ariel and in 2011 affiliation with Center for Pediatric Chronic Diseases and Center for Down Syndrome, Department of Pediatrics, Hadassah-Hebrew University Medical Center, Mount Scopus Campus, Jerusalem.

International collaborations

Internationally with the Department of Disability and Human Development, College of Applied Health Sciences, University of Illinois at Chicago; Strong Center for Developmental Disabilities, Golisano Children's Hospital at Strong, University of Rochester School of Medicine and Dentistry, New York; Centre on Intellectual Disabilities, University of Albany, New York; Centre for Chronic Disease Prevention and Control, Health Canada, Ottawa; Chandler Medical Center and Children's Hospital, Kentucky Children's Hospital, Section of Adolescent Medicine, University of Kentucky, Lexington; Chronic Disease Prevention and

Control Research Center, Baylor College of Medicine, Houston, Texas; Division of Neuroscience, Department of Psychiatry, Columbia University, New York; Institute for the Study of Disadvantage and Disability, Atlanta; Center for Autism and Related Disorders, Department Psychiatry, Children's Hospital Boston, Boston; Department of Paediatrics, Child Health and Adolescent Medicine, Children's Hospital at Westmead, Westmead, Australia; International Centre for the Study of Occupational and Mental Health, Düsseldorf, Germany; Centre for Advanced Studies in Nursing, Department of General Practice and Primary Care, University of Aberdeen, Aberdeen, United Kingdom; Quality of Life Research Center, Copenhagen, Denmark; Nordic School of Public Health, Gottenburg, Sweden, Scandinavian Institute of Quality of Working Life, Oslo, Norway; Centre for Quality of Life of the Hong Kong Institute of Asia-Pacific Studies and School of Social Work, Chinese University, Hong Kong.

Targets

Our focus is on research, international collaborations, clinical work, teaching and policy in health, disability and human development and to establish the NICHD as a permanent institute at one of the residential care centers for persons with intellectual disability in Israel in order to conduct model research and together with the four university schools of public health/medicine in Israel establish a national master and doctoral program in disability and human development at the institute to secure the next generation of professionals working in this often non-prestigious/low-status field of work.

Contact

Joav Merrick, MD, DMSc

Professor of Pediatrics, Child Health and Human Development

Medical Director, Health Services, Division for Intellectual and Developmental Disabilities, Ministry of Social Affairs and Social Services, POB 1260, IL-91012 Jerusalem, Israel.

E-mail: jmerrick@inter.net.il

Chapter 17

About the book series "Pediatrics, child and adolescent health"

Pediatrics, child and adolescent health is a book series with publications from a multidisciplinary group of researchers, practitioners and clinicians for an international professional forum interested in the broad spectrum of pediatric medicine, child health, adolescent health and human development.

- Merrick J, ed. Child and adolescent health yearbook 2011. New York: Nova Science, 2012.
- Merrick J, ed. Child and adolescent health yearbook 2012. New York: Nova Science, 2012.
- Roach RR, Greydanus DE, Patel DR, Homnick DN, Merrick J, eds. Tropical pediatrics: A public health concern of international proportions. New York: Nova Science, 2012.
- Merrick J, ed. Child health and human development yearbook 2011. New York: Nova Science, 2012.
- Merrick J, ed. Child health and human development yearbook 2012. New York: Nova Science, 2012.

Contact

Professor Joav Merrick, MD, MMedSci, DMSc
Medical Director, Medical Services
Division for Intellectual and Developmental Disabilities
Ministry of Social Affairs and Social Services
POBox 1260
IL-91012 Jerusalem, Israel
E-mail: jmerrick@zahav.net.il
Home-page: http://jmerrick50.googlepages.com/home

Index

D

E

F

G

H

I

J

K

L

M

N

O

P

Q

R

S

W

Y